Cultural Diversity in Health and Illness

CUSTOM EDITION FOR ROSS
EDUCATION

Rachel E. Spector

Taken From:

Cultural Diversity in Health and Illness, Seventh Edition
by Rachel E. Spector

Learning Solutions

New York   Boston   San Francisco
London   Toronto   Sydney   Tokyo   Singapore   Madrid
Mexico City   Munich   Paris   Cape Town   Hong Kong   Montreal

Cover Art: Courtesy of Digitalvision, PhotoDisc/Getty Images.

Taken from:

Cultural Diversity in Health and Illness, Seventh Edition
by Rachel E. Spector
Copyright © 2009 by Pearson Education, Inc.
Published by Prentice Hall
Upper Saddle River, NJ 07458

This special edition published in cooperation with Pearson Learning Solutions.

Pearson Learning Solutions, 501 Boylston Street, Suite 900, Boston, MA 02116
A Pearson Education Company
www.pearsoned.com

Printed in the United States of America

21

ST

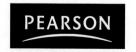

ISBN 10: 0-558-81714-9
ISBN 13: 978-0-558-81714-5

I would like to dedicate this text to

My husband, Manny;
Sam, Hilary, Julia, and Emma;
Becky, Perry, Naomi, Rose, and Miriam;
the memory of my parents, Joseph J. and Freda F. Needleman,
and my in-laws, Sam and Margaret Spector;
and the memory of my beloved mentor, Irving Kenneth Zola.

Contents

Preface

In 1977—more than 30 years ago—I prepared the first edition of *Cultural Diversity in Health and Illness*. Now, as I begin the seventh edition of this book—the sixth revision—I realize that this is an opportunity to reflect on an endeavor that has filled a good deal of my life for the past 30 years. I believe this book has a soul and it, in turn, has become an integral part of my soul. I have lived—through practice, teaching, and research—this material since 1974 and have developed many ways of presenting this content. In addition, I have tracked for 30 years

1. The United States Census
2. Immigration—numbers and policies
3. Poverty—figures and policies
4. Health care—costs and policies
5. Morbidity and mortality rates
6. Nursing and other health care manpower issues

My metaphors are *HEALTH*, defined as "the balance of the person, both within one's being—physical, mental, and spiritual—and in the outside world—natural, communal, and metaphysical"; *ILLNESS*, the imbalance of the person, both within one's being—physical, mental, and spiritual—and in the outside world—natural, communal, and metaphysical; and *HEALING*, the restoration of balance, both within one's being—physical, mental, and spiritual—and in the outside world—natural, communal, and metaphysical." I have learned over these years that within many traditional heritages (defined as "old," not contemporary or modern) people tend to define HEALTH, ILLNESS, and HEALING in this manner. Imagine a kaleidoscope—the tube can represent HEALTH. The objects reflected within the kaleidoscope reflect the traditional tools used to care for a given person's HEALTH. If you love kaleidoscopes, you know what I am describing and that the patterns that emerge are infinite.

In addition, I have had the unique opportunity to travel to countless places in the United States and abroad. I make it a practice to visit the traditional mar-

kets, pharmacies, and shrines and dialogue with the people who work in or patron-
ize the settings and have gathered invaluable knowledge and unique items and images. My tourist dollars are invested in amulets and remedies and my collection is
large. Digital photography has changed my eyes; I may be a "digital immigrant,"
rather than a "digital native," but the camera has proven to be my most treasured
companion. I have been able to use the images of sacred objects and sacred places
to create HEALTH Traditions Imagery. The opening images for each chapter and
countless images within the chapters are the results of these explorations. Given
that there are times when we do not completely understand a concept or an image, several images are slightly blurred or dark to represent this wonderment.

The first edition of this book was the outcome of a *promesa*—a promise—
I once made. The promise was made to a group of Asian, Black, and Hispanic
students I taught in a medical sociology course in 1973. In this course, the students wound up being the teachers, and they taught me to see the world of
health care delivery through the eyes of the health care consumer rather than
through my own well-intentioned eyes. What I came to see I did not always like.
I did not realize how much I did not know; I believed I knew a lot. I promised
the students that I would take that which they taught me regarding HEALTH and
teach it to students and colleagues. I have held on to the *promesa*, and my experiences over the years have been incredible. I have met people and traveled. At
all times I have held on to the idea and goal of attempting to help nurses and
other health care providers be aware of and sensitive to the HEALTH, ILLNESS, and
HEALING beliefs and needs of their patients.

I know that looking inside closed doors carries with it a risk. I know that
people prefer to think that our society is a melting pot and that the traditional
beliefs and practices have vanished with the expected acculturation and assimilation into mainstream North American modern life. Many people, however, have
continued to carry on the traditional customs and culture from their native lands
and heritage, and HEALTH, ILLNESS, and HEALING beliefs are deeply entwined
within the cultural and social beliefs that people have. To understand HEALTH
and ILLNESS beliefs and practices, it is necessary to see each person in his or her
unique sociocultural world. The theoretical knowledge that has evolved for the
development of this text is cumulative and much of the "old" material is relevant today as many HEALTH, ILLNESS, and HEALING beliefs do not change. However, many beliefs and practices do go underground.

The purpose of each edition has been to increase awareness of the dimensions and complexities involved in caring for people from diverse cultural backgrounds. I wished to share my personal experiences and thoughts concerning
the introduction of cultural concepts into the education of health care professionals. The books represented my answers to the questions:

■ "How does one effectively expose a student to cultural diversity?"
■ "How does one examine health care issues and perceptions from a broad
social viewpoint?"

As I have done in the classroom, I attempt to bring you, the reader, into direct contact with the interaction between providers of care within the North American health care system and the consumers of health care. The staggering issues of health care delivery are explored and contrasted with the choices that people may make in attempting to deal with health care issues.

It is now imperative, according to the most recent policies of the Joint Commission of Hospital Accreditation and the Centers for Medicare & Medicaid Services, that all health care providers be "culturally competent." In this context, cultural competency implies that within the delivery of care the health care provider understands and attends to the total context of the patient's situation; it is a complex combination of knowledge, attitudes, and skills, yet

- How do you *really* inspire people to hear the content?
- How do you *motivate* providers to see the worldview and lived experience of the patient?
- How do you assist providers to *really* bear witness to the living conditions and life ways of patients?
- How do you liberate providers from the burdens of prejudice, xenophobia, the "isms"—racism, ethnocentrism—and the "antis"?

It can be argued that the development of CULTURALCOMPETENCY does not occur in a short encounter with cultural diversity but that it takes time to develop the skills, knowledge, and attitudes to safely and satisfactorily deliver CULTURALCARE. Indeed, the reality of becoming "CULTURALCOMPETENT" is a complex process—it is time consuming, difficult, frustrating, and extremely interesting. CULTURALCOMPETENCY embraces the premise that all things are connected. Imagine a dandelion that has gone to seed. Each seed is a discrete entity, yet each is linked to the other (Figure P–1). Each facet discussed in this text—heritage, culture, ethnicity, religion, socialization, and identity—is connected to diversity—demographic change—population, immigration, and poverty. These facets are connected to health/HEALTH, illness/ILLNESS, curing/HEALING, and beliefs and practices, modern and traditional. All of these facets are connected to the health care delivery system—the culture, costs, and politics of health care, the internal and external political issues, public health issues, and housing and other infrastructure issues. In order to fully understand a person's health/HEALTH beliefs and practices, each of these topics must be in the background of a provider's mind.

I have had the opportunity to live and teach in Spain and to explore many areas, including Cadiz and the surrounding small villages. There was a fake door within the walls of a small village, *Vejer de la Frontera* (Figure P–2), that appeared to be bolted shut. The door was placed there during the early 14th century to fool the Barbary pirates. The people were able to vanquish them while they tried to pry the door open. It reminded me of the attempt to keep other ideas and people away from us and to not open ourselves up to new and different ideas. Another door (Figure P–3), found in Avila, Spain, was made of a translucent glass. Here, the person has a choice—you could peer through the door and view the garden behind it or open it and actually go into the garden

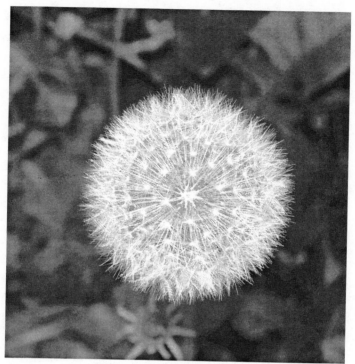

Figure P-1   A dandelion in seed.

for a finite walk. This reminded me of people who are able to understand the needs of others and return to their own life and heritage when work is completed. This polarity represents the challenges of "CULTURALCOMPETENCY."

The way to CULTURALCOMPETENCY is complex, but I have learned over the years that there are five steps (Figure P–4) to climb to begin to achieve this goal:

1. Personal heritage—Who are *you*?? What is *your* heritage? What are your health/HEALTH beliefs?
2. Heritage of others—demographics—Who is the patient? Family? Community?
3. Health and HEALTH beliefs and practices—competing philosophies
4. Health care culture and system—all the issues and problems
5. Traditional HEALTH Care Systems—The way HEALTH was for most and the way HEALTH still is for many

Once you have reached the sixth step, CULTURALCOMPETENCY, you are ready to open the door to CULTURALCARE.

Each step represents a discrete unit of study. The steps are composed of "bricks" and these provide the ingredients for the content. The "bricks" are

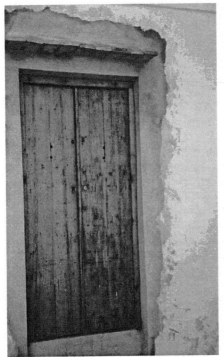

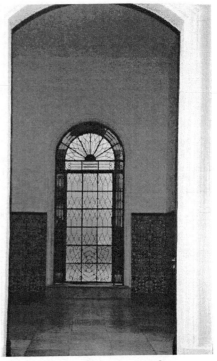

Figure P-2   Solidly closed door.   **Figure P-3   Transparent door.**

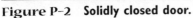

defined in the glossary, Appendix A and are the language of CULTURALCARE. The side rails represent responsibility and resiliency—for it is the responsibility of health care providers to be CULTURALLYCOMPETENT and, if this is not met, the consequences will be dire. The resiliency of providers and patients will be further compromised and we will all become more vulnerable. Contrary to popular belief and practice, CULTURALCOMPETENCY is not a "condition" that is rapidly achieved. Rather, it is an ongoing process of growth and the development of knowledge that takes a considerable amount of time to ingest, digest, assimilate, circulate, and master. The content is readily available:

- Countless books and articles have been published in nursing, medicine, public health, and the popular media over the past 40 years that contain invaluable information relevant to CULTURALCOMPETENCY.
- Innumerable workshops and meetings have been available where the content is presented and discussed.
- "Self-study" programs on the Internet have been developed that provide continuing education credits to nurses, physicians, and other providers.

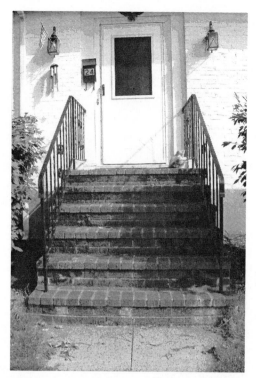

Figure P-4   The steps to CULTURALCOMPETENCY.

However, the process of becoming CULTURALLYCOMPETENT is not generally provided for. Issues persist, such as

▩ Demographic disparity exists in the profile of health care providers and in health status.

▩ Patient needs, such as modesty, space, and gender-specific care, are not universally met.

▩ Religious-specific needs are not met in terms of meal planning, procedural planning, conference planning, and so forth.

▩ Communication and language barriers exist.

As this knowledge is built, you are on the way to CULTURALCOMPETENCY. As it matures and grows, you become an advocate of CULTURALCARE, as it will be described in Chapter 1.

This book has been developed to provide an overview of the information necessary to climb these steps and examples of the process.

Supplemental Resources

■ **CulturalCare Guide.** Previously available as a separate booklet, the contents of this helpful guide are now available for downloading on the Companion Website. The guide includes the Heritage Assessment Tool, Cultural Phenomena Affecting Health Care, CulturalCare Etiquette, and other assessment tools and guides.

■ **Companion Website.** www.prenhall.com/spector. The Companion Website includes a wealth of supplemental material to accompany each chapter. In addition to the complete contents of the **CulturalCare Guide**, the site presents chapter-related review questions, case studies, exercises, and MediaLinks to provide additional information. Panorama of Health and Illness videos accompany many chapters, and a glossary of terms appears for each chapter. Also included is a collection of the author's photographs and culturally significant images in the **CulturalCare Museum**.

■ **Instructor's Resource Center.** Available to instructors adopting the book are PowerPoint Lecture Slides and a complete testbank available for downloading from the Instructor's Resource Center, which can be accessed through the online catalog.

■ **Online Course Management.** Built to accompany *Cultural Diversity in Health and Illness* are online course management systems available for Blackboard, WebCT, Moodle, Angel, and other platforms. For more information, contact your Pearson Education sales representative.

About the Author

Dr. Rachel E. Spector has been a student of culturally diverse HEALTH and ILLNESS beliefs and practices for 35 years and has researched and taught courses on culture and HEALTH care for the same time span. Dr. Spector has had the opportunity to work in many different communities, including the American Indian and Hispanic communities in Boston, Massachusetts. Her studies have taken her to many places: most of the United States, Canada, and Mexico; several European countries, including Denmark, England, Finland, Iceland, Italy, France, Russia, Spain, and Switzerland; Israel and Pakistan; and Australia and New Zealand. She was fortunate enough to collect traditional amulets and remedies from many of these diverse communities and to meet practitioners of traditional HEALTH care in several places. She was instrumental in the creation and presentation of the exhibit "Immigrant HEALTH Traditions" at the Ellis Island Immigration Museum, May 1994 through January 1995. She has exhibited HEALTH-related objects in several other settings. Recently, she served as a *Colaboradora Honorifica* (Honorary Collaborator) in the University of Alicante in Alicante, Spain, and Tamaulipas, Mexico. In 2006, she was a Lady Davis Fellow in the Henrietta Zold-Hadassah Hebrew University School of Nursing in Jerusalem, Israel. This text was translated into Spanish by Maria Munoz and published in Madrid by Prentice Hall as *Las Culturas de la SALUD* in 2003. She is a Fellow in the American Academy of Nursing and a Scholar in Transcultural Nursing. The Massachusetts Association of Registered Nurses, the state organization of the American Nurses' Association, honored her as a "Living Legend" in 2007. In 2008 she received the Honorary Human Rights Award from the American Nurses Association. This award recognized her contributions and accomplishments that have been of national significance to human rights and have influenced health care and nursing practice.

Acknowledgments

I have had a 35-year adventure of studying the forces of culture, ethnicity, and religion and their profound influence on HEALTH, ILLNESS, and HEALING beliefs and practices. Many, many people have contributed generously to the knowledge I have acquired over this time as I have tried to serve as a voice for traditional people and the HEALTH, ILLNESS, and HEALING beliefs and practices derived from their given heritage. It has been a continuous struggle to insure that this information be included not only in nursing education but in the educational content of all helping professions—including medicine, the allied health professions, and social work.

I particularly wish to thank the following people for their guidance, professional support, and encouragement over the 32 years that this book, now in its seventh edition, has been an integral part of my life. They are people from many walks of life and have touched me in many ways. The people from Appleton-Century-Crofts, which became Appleton & Lang and then became Prentice Hall. They include Nancy Anselment, Sally Barhydt, Dave Caroll, Elisabeth Garafalo, Marion Kalstein-Welch, Pamela Lappies, Cathy O'Connell, Julie Stern, Patrick Walsh, and countless people involved in the production of the text. My first encounter with publishing was with Leslie Boyer, an acquisition editor from Appleton-Century-Crofts, who simply said "write a book" in 1976. For this edition I have worked closely with Michael Giacobbe, development editor, as not only an editor but a friend, a cheerleader, an encourager, and so forth. Without his patient help and guidance, this book would not be here today. Thanks to Teresa O'Neill of Our Lady of Holy Cross College for writing chapter review questions. The many people who helped with advice and guidance to resources over the years include Elsi Basque, Billye Brown, Louise Buchanan, Julian Castillo, Leonel J. Castillo, Jenny Chan, Dr. P. K. Chan, Joe Colorado, Miriam Cook, Elizabeth Cucchiaro, Mary A. Dineen, Norine Dresser, Celeste Dye, Laverne Gallman, Raymond and Madeline Goodman, Marjory Gordon, Orlando Isaza, Henry and Pandora Law, Hawk Littlejohn, Father Richard McCabe, S. Dale McLemore, Anita Noble, Carl Rutberg, Sister Mary Nicholas Vincelli, Nora Wang, David Warner, Ann Marie Yezzi-Shareef, and the late Irving K. Zola.

I wish to thank my friends and family, who have tolerated my absence at numerous social functions, and the many people who have provided the numerous support services necessary for the completion of an undertaking such as this.

A lot has happened in my life since the first edition of this book was published in 1979. My family has shrunk with the deaths of all four parents, and it has greatly expanded with a new daughter, Hilary, and a new son, Perry, and five granddaughters—Julia, Emma, Naomi, Rose, and Miriam. The generations have gone, and come.

Reviewers

Michelle Gagnon, BS, RUT, RDCS
Bunker Hill Community College
Boston, MA

Marie Gates, PhD
WMU Bronson School of Nursing
Kalamazoo, MI

Janette McCrory, MSN
Delta State University
Cleveland, MS

Anita Noble, DNSc
Henrietta Zold-Hadassah Hebrew University School of Nursing
Jerusalem, Israel

A Word About HEALTH

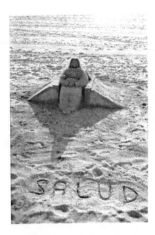

Sand Sculpture—Postiquet Beach, Alicante, Spain

HEALTH connotes the balance of a person, both within one's being—physical, mental, and spiritual—and in the outside world—natural, familial and communal, and metaphysical. The model is a method for describing beliefs and practices used to **maintain** through daily HEALTH practices, such as diet, activities, and clothing; to **protect** through special HEALTH practices, such as food taboos, seasonal activities, and protective items worn, carried, or hung in the home or workplace; and/or to **restore** through special HEALTH practices, such as diet changes, rest, special clothing or objects, **physical, mental, and/or spiritual** HEALTH. The accompanying image, *SALUD*, is a metaphor for HEALTH in countless ways. Here, it is whole and emerging from the shadows of early morning. Just as the sand sculpture is fragile, disappearing overnight, so, too, is HEALTH. It brings to mind the reality that each of us has the internal responsibility to maintain, protect, and restore our HEALTH; the reciprocal holds true for the external familial, environmental, and societal forces—they, too, must look after and safeguard our HEALTH. This book, in part, is a mirror that reflects the countless ways by which people are able to maintain, protect, and/or restore their HEALTH. Just as there is an interplay between a sand sculpture and the natural forces that can create and harm and destroy it, so, too, it is with HEALTH and the forces of the outside world.

ILLNESS is the imbalance of the person, both within one's being—physical, mental, and spiritual—and in the outside world—natural, familial and communal, and metaphysical. HEALING is the restoration of this balance. The relationships of the person to the outside world are reciprocal.

When these terms, HEALTH, ILLNESS, AND HEALING are used in small capitals in this text, it is to connote that they are being used holistically. When they are written *health, illness,* and *healing,* they are to be understood in the common way.

The cover uses the sculpture as its focal point surrounded by selected segments of HEALTH related images. The segments are from the opening images of several chapters of this book and the explanations for each image can be found in the opening paragraphs of the chapters.

Cultural Diversity
in Health and Illness

Unit

I

Cultural Foundations

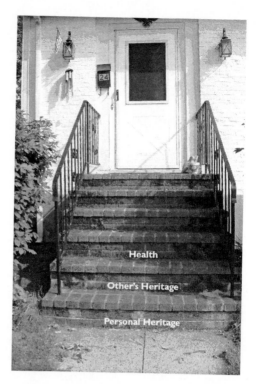

Unit I creates the foundation for this book and enables you to become aware of the importance of cultural heritage and history—both your own and those of other people; the importance of understanding diversity—demographic, immigration, and economic—and importance of the standard concepts of health and illness.

Before you read Unit I, please answer the following questions:

1. What is your sociocultural heritage?
2. What major sociocultural events have occurred in your lifetime?
3. What is the demographic profile of the community you grew up in? How has it changed?
4. How would you acquire economic help if necessary?
5. How do you define *health*?
6. How do you define *illness*?
7. What do you do to maintain your health?
8. What do you do to protect your health?
9. What do you do when you experience a noticeable change in your health?
10. Do you diagnose your own health problems? If yes, how do you do so? If no, why not?
11. From whom do you seek health care?
12. What do you do to restore your health? Give examples.

1

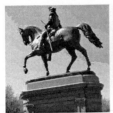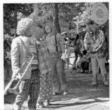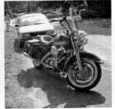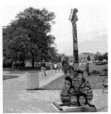

Chapter 1

Cultural Heritage and History

When there is a very dense cultural barrier, you do the best you can, and if something happens despite that, you have to be satisfied with little success instead of total successes. You have to give up total control. . . .

—Anne Fadiman (1997)

■ Objectives

1. Describe the National Standards for Culturally and Linguistically Appropriate Services in Health Care.
2. Articulate the attributes of CulturalCompetency and CULTURALCARE.
3. Explain the factors involved in the cultural phenomena affecting health.

In all clinical practice areas—from institutional settings, such as acute and long-term care settings, to community-based settings, such as nurse practitioner's and doctor's offices and clinics, schools and universities, public health, and occupational settings—one observes diversity every day. The compelling need for culturally and linguistically competent health care services for diverse populations has attracted increased attention from health care providers and those who judge their quality and efficiency for many years. The mainstream health care provider is treating a more diverse patient population as a result of demographic changes and participation in insurance programs, and the interest in designing culturally and linguistically appropriate services that lead to improved health care outcomes, efficiency, and patient satisfaction has increased.

One's personal cultural background, heritage, and language have a considerable impact on both how patients access and respond to health care services and how the providers practice within the system. **Cultural** and **linguistic competence** suggests an ability by health care providers and health care organizations to understand and respond effectively to the cultural and linguistic needs brought to the health care experience. This is a phenomenon that recognizes the diversity that exists among the patients, physicians, nurses, and caregivers. This phenomenon is not limited to the changes in the patient population in that it also embraces the members of the workforce—including providers from other countries. Many of the people in the workforce are new immigrants and/or are from ethnocultural backgrounds that are different from that of the dominant culture.

In addition, health and illness can be interpreted and explained in terms of personal experience and expectations. We can define our own health or illness and determine what these states mean to us in our daily lives. We learn from our own cultural and ethnic backgrounds how to be healthy, how to recognize illness, and how to be ill. Furthermore, the meanings we attach to the notions of health and illness are related to the basic, culture-bound values by which we define a given experience and perception.

This first chapter presents an overview of the salient content and complex theoretical content related to one's heritage and their impact on health beliefs and practices. Two sets of theories are presented, the first of which analyzes the degree to which people have maintained their traditional heritage; the second, and opposite, set of theories relates to socialization and acculturation and the quasi creation of a melting pot or some other common threads that are part of an American whole. It then becomes possible to analyze health beliefs by determining a person's ties to his or her traditional heritage, rather than to signs of acculturation. The assumption is that there is a relationship between people with strong identities—either with their heritage or the level at which they are acculturated into the American culture—and their health beliefs and practices. Hand in hand with the concept of ethnocultural heritage is that of a person's ethnocultural history, the journey a person has experienced predicated on the historical sociocultural events that have touched his or her life directly or indirectly.

Box 1–1

National Standards for Culturally and Linguistically Appropriate Services in Health Care

1. Health care organizations should ensure that patients/consumers receive from all staff members effective, understandable, and respectful care that is provided in a manner compatible with their cultural health beliefs and practices and preferred language.
2. Health care organizations should implement strategies to recruit, retain, and promote at all levels of the organization a diverse staff and leadership that are representative of the demographic characteristics of the service area.
3. Health care organizations should ensure that staff at all levels and across all disciplines receive ongoing education and training in culturally and linguistically appropriate service delivery.
4. Health care organizations must offer and provide language assistance services, including bilingual staff and interpreter services, at no cost to each patient/consumer with limited English proficiency at all points of contact, in a timely manner during all hours of operation.
5. Health care organizations must provide to patients/consumers in their preferred language both verbal offers and written notices informing them of their right to receive language assistance services.
6. Health care organizations must assure the competence of language assistance provided to limited English-proficient patients/consumers by interpreters and bilingual staff. Family and friends should not be used to provide interpretation services (except on request by the patient/consumer).
7. Health care organizations must make available easily understood patient-related materials and post signage in the languages of the commonly encountered groups and/or groups represented in the service area.
8. Health care organizations should develop, implement, and promote a written strategic plan that outlines clear goals, policies, operational plans, and management accountability/oversight mechanisms to provide culturally and linguistically appropriate services.
9. Health care organizations should conduct initial and ongoing organizational self-assessments of CLAS-related activities and are encouraged to integrate cultural and linguistic competence– related measures into their internal audits, performance improvement programs, patient satisfaction assessments, and outcomes-based evaluations.
10. Health care organizations should ensure that data on the individual patient's/ consumer's race, ethnicity, and spoken and written language are collected in health records, integrated into the organization's management information systems, and periodically updated.
11. Health care organizations should maintain a current demographic, cultural, and epidemiological profile of the community as well as a needs assessment

to accurately plan for and implement services that respond to the cultural and linguistic characteristics of the service area.

12. Health care organizations should develop participatory, collaborative partnerships with communities and utilize a variety of formal and informal mechanisms to facilitate community and patient/consumer involvement in designing and implementing CLAS-related activities.

13. Health care organizations should ensure that conflict and grievance resolution processes are culturally and linguistically sensitive and capable of identifying, preventing, and resolving cross-cultural conflicts or complaints by patients/consumers.

14. Health care organizations are encouraged to regularly make available to the public information about their progress and successful innovations in implementing the CLAS standards and to provide public notice in their communities about the availability of this information.

Source: National Standards for Culturally and Linguistically Appropriate Services in Health Care. Final Report. Washington, DC, March 2001. For full report and discussion, contact the Office of Minority Health: Guadalupe Pacheco, MSW, Special Assistant to the Director, Project Officer, Office of Minority Health, Office of Public Health and Science, U.S. Department of Health and Human Services, Rockwall II, Suite 1000, 5515 Security Lane, Rockville, MD 20852, phone: 301-443-5084, gpacheco@osophs.dhhs.gov.

National Standards for Culturally and Linguistically Appropriate Services in Health Care

In 1997, the Office of Minority Health undertook the development of national standards to provide a much needed alternative to the patchwork that has been undertaken in the field of Cultural Diversity. It developed the National Standards for Culturally and Linguistically Appropriate Services (CLAS) in Health Care. These 14 standards (Box 1-1) must be met by most health care–related agencies. The standards are based on an analytical review of key laws, regulations, contracts, and standards currently in use by federal and state agencies and other national organizations. They were developed with input from a national advisory committee of policymakers, health care providers, and researchers.

Accreditation and credentialing agencies can assess and compare providers who say they provide culturally competent services and assure quality care for diverse populations. This includes the Joint Commission on Accreditation of Healthcare Organizations (JCAHO); the National Committee on Quality Assurance; professional organizations, such as the American Medical and Nurses Associations; and quality review organizations, such as peer review organizations.

In order to ensure both equal access to quality health care by diverse populations and a secure work environment, all health care providers must "promote and support the attitudes, behaviors, knowledge, and skills necessary for staff to work respectfully and effectively with patients and each other in a culturally diverse work environment" (Office of Minority Health, 2001, p. 7). This is the first and fundamental standard of the 14 standards that have been recommended as national standards for culturally and linguistically appropriate services (CLAS) in health care.

■ Cultural Competence

Cultural competence implies that professional health care must be developed to be culturally sensitive, culturally appropriate, and culturally competent. Culturally Competent Care is critical to meet the complex culture-bound health care needs of a given person, family, and community. It is the provision of health care across cultural boundaries and takes into account the context in which the patient lives, as well as the situations in which the patient's health problems arise.

- ■ **Culturally competent**—within the delivered care, the provider understands and attends to the total context of the patient's situation and this is a complex combination of knowledge, attitudes, and skills.
- ■ **Culturally appropriate**—the provider applies the underlying background knowledge that must be possessed to provide a patient with the best possible health/HEALTH care.
- ■ **Culturally sensitive**—the provider possesses some basic knowledge of and constructive attitudes toward the health/HEALTH traditions observed among the diverse cultural groups found in the setting in which he or she is practicing.

■ Linguistic Competence

Linguistic competence embraces the concept of linguistically appropriate services and espouses the implementation of competent interpreter services when the patient and family do not understand, speak, or read English. Under the provisions of Title VI of the Civil Rights Act of 1964, people with Limited English Proficiency (LEP) who are cared for in both institutional and community health facilities, such as

- ■ Hospitals
- ■ Day care centers
- ■ Mental health centers
- ■ Senior citizen centers
- ■ Family health centers and clinics

and are eligible for Medicaid, other health care, or human services cannot be denied assistance because of their race, color, or national origin. There are many forms of illegal discrimination that frequently limit the opportunities of people to gain equal access to health care services. The language barriers experienced by Limited English Proficiency (LEP) persons can result in limiting access to critical public health, hospital, and other medical and social services.

▓ CULTURALCARE

The term *CULTURALCARE* expresses all that is inherent in the development of health care delivery to meet the mandates of the CLAS standards, and CULTURAL-CARE is holistic. There are countless conflicts in the health care delivery arenas that are predicated on cultural misunderstandings. Although many of these misunderstandings are related to universal situations—such as verbal and nonverbal language misunderstandings, the conventions of courtesy, the sequencing of interactions, the phasing of interactions, and objectivity—many cultural misunderstandings are unique to the delivery of health care. The need to provide CULTURALCARE is essential, and providers must be able to assess and interpret a patient's health beliefs and practices and cultural needs. CULTURALCARE alters the perspective of health care delivery as it enables the provider to understand, from a cultural perspective, the manifestations of the patient's cultural heritage and life trajectory. The provider must serve as a bridge in the health care setting between the patient and people who are from different cultural backgrounds.

▓ Cultural Phenomena Affecting Health

Giger and Davidhizar (1995) have identified six cultural phenomena that vary among cultural groups and affect health care: environmental control, biological variations, social organization, communication, space, and time orientation.

Environmental Control

Environmental control is the ability of members of a particular cultural group to plan activities that control nature or direct environmental factors. Included in this concept are the complex systems of traditional health and illness beliefs, the practice of folk medicine, and the use of traditional healers. This cultural phenomenon plays an extremely important role in the way patients respond to health-related experiences, including the ways in which they define *health* and *illness* and seek and use health care resources and social supports.

Biological Variations

The several ways in which people from one cultural group differ biologically (i.e., physically and genetically) from members of other cultural groups constitute their biological variations. The following are significant examples:

- ▓ Body build and structure, including specific bone and structural differences between groups, such as the smaller stature of Asians
- ▓ Skin color, including variations in tone, texture, healing abilities, and hair follicles
- ▓ Enzymatic and genetic variations, including differences in response to drug and dietary therapies

■ Susceptibility to disease, which can manifest as a higher morbidity rate of certain diseases within certain groups

■ Nutritional variations, countless examples of which include the "hot and cold" preferences among Hispanic Americans, the yin and yang preferences among Asian Americans, and the rules of the kosher diet among Jewish and Islamic Americans; a relatively common nutritional disorder, lactose intolerance, is found among Mexican, African, Asian, and Eastern European Jewish Americans

Social Organization

The social environment in which people grow up and live plays an essential role in their cultural development and identification. Children learn their culture's responses to life events from the family and its ethnoreligious group. This socialization process is an inherent part of heritage—cultural, religious, and ethnic background. *Social organization* refers to the family unit (nuclear, single-parent, or extended family) and the *social group organizations* (religious or ethnic) with which patients and families may identify. Countless social barriers, such as unemployment, underemployment, homelessness, lack of health insurance, and poverty, can also prevent people from entering the health care system.

Communication

Communication differences present themselves in many ways, including language differences, verbal and nonverbal behaviors, and silence. Language differences are possibly the most important obstacle to providing multicultural health care because they affect all stages of the patient-caregiver relationship. Clear and effective communication is important when dealing with any patient, especially if language differences create a cultural barrier. When deprived of the most common medium of interaction with patients—the spoken word—health care providers often become frustrated and ineffective. Accurate diagnosis and treatment is impossible if the health care professional cannot understand the patient. When the provider is not understood, he or she often avoids verbal communication and does not realize the effect of nonverbal communication, which is all too often the painful isolation of patients who do not speak the dominant language and who are in an unfamiliar environment. Consequently, patients experience cultural shock and may react by withdrawing, becoming hostile or belligerent, or being uncooperative.

Language differences can be bridged, however, with the use of competent interpreters. If the patient does not speak the dominant language, a skilled interpreter is mandatory.

Space

Personal space refers to people's behaviors and attitudes toward the space around themselves. Territoriality is the behavior and attitude people exhibit about an area they have claimed and defend or react emotionally about when others encroach on it. Both personal space and territoriality are influenced by culture, and thus different ethnocultural groups have varying norms related to the use of space. Space and related behaviors have different meanings in the following zones:

- Intimate zone—extends up to 1½ feet. Because this distance allows adults to have the most bodily contact for perception of breath and odor, incursion into this zone is acceptable only in private places. Visual distortions also occur at this distance.

- Personal distance—extends from 1½ to 4 feet. This is an extension of the self that is like having a "bubble" of space surrounding the body. At this distance, the voice may be moderate, body odor may not be apparent, and visual distortion may have disappeared.

- Social distance—extends from 4 to 12 feet. This is reserved for impersonal business transactions. Perceptual information is much less detailed.

- Public distance—extends 12 feet or more. Individuals interact only impersonally. Communicators' voices must be projected, and subtle facial expressions may be lost.

It must be noted that these generalizations about the use of personal space are based on studies of the behavior of European North Americans. The use of personal space varies among individuals and ethnic groups. The extreme modesty practiced by members of some cultural groups may prevent members from seeking preventive health care.

Time Orientation

The viewing of time in the present, past, or future varies among cultural groups. Certain cultures in the United States and Canada tend to be future-oriented. People who are future-oriented are concerned with long-range goals and with health care measures in the present to prevent the occurrence of illness in the future. They prefer to plan by making schedules, setting appointments, and organizing activities. Others are oriented more to the present than the future and may be late for appointments because they are less concerned about planning to be on time. This difference in time orientation may become important in health care measures such as long-term planning and explanations of medication schedules.

Figure 1–1 illustrates how a person, with a unique ethnic, religious, and cultural background, is affected by cultural phenomena. The discussions in Chapters 6 through 10 highlight these phenomena, and examples are presented within the text and in tabular form. The examples used in the text to illustrate

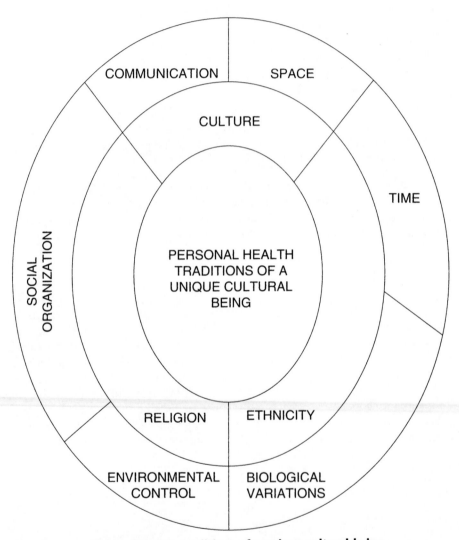

Figure 1-1 Personal health traditions of a unique cultural being.

Table 1-1   Examples of Etiquette as Related to Selected Cultural Phenomena

Time	Visiting Being on time Taboo times	Inform person when you are coming Avoid surprises Explain your expectations about time Ask people from other regions and cultures what they expect Be familiar with the times and meanings of person's ethnic and religious holidays
Space	Body language and distances	Know cultural and/or religious customs regarding contact, such as eye and touch, from many perspectives
Communication	Greetings Gestures Smiling Eye contact	Know the proper forms of address for people from a given culture and the ways by which people welcome one another Know when touch, such as an embrace or a handshake, is expected and when physical contact is prohibited Gestures do not have universal meaning; what is acceptable to one cultural group is taboo with another Smiles may be indicative of friendliness to some, taboo to others Avoiding eye contact may be a sign of respect
Social organization	Holidays Special events Births Weddings Funerals	Know what dates are important and why, whether to give gifts, what to wear to special events, and what the customs and beliefs are Know how the event is celebrated, the meaning of colors used for gifts, and expected rituals at home or religious services
Biological variations	Food customs	Know what can be eaten for certain events, what foods may be eaten together or are forbidden, and what and how utensils are used
Environmental control	Health practices and remedies	Know what the general HEALTH traditions are for person and question observations for validity

Source: Adapted from Dresser, N. (1996). *Multicultural manners*. New York: Wiley. Copyright ©1996 John Wiley & Sons, Inc. Reprinted by permission of John Wiley & Sons. Inc.

health traditions in different cultures are not intended to be stereotypical. With careful listening, observing, and questioning, the provider should be able to sort out the traditions of a given person. Table 1–1 suggests examples of etiquette relevant to each of the cultural phenomena.

This chapter has served as the foundation that delineates the multiple, interrelating phenomena that underlie the cultural conflict that occurs between health care providers and patients, many of whom have difficulty interacting with the health care providers and system. It has presented both classical and contemporary definitions and explanations relevant to the foundation of this conflict and sets the stage for further discussion.

Explore 🌐 MediaLink

Go to the Companion Website at www.prenhall.com/spector for chapter-related review questions, case studies, and activities. Contents of the CulturalCare Guide and CulturalCare Museum can also be found on the Companion Website. Click on Chapter 1 to select the activities for this chapter.

▓ Internet Sources

Kohut, A., and Rogers, M. (2002) Americans Struggle with Religion's Role at Home and Abroad. Washington, DC: Pew Research Center. Retrieved from http://www.adherents.com/rel_USA.html. July 22, 2007.

Kohut, A., and Rogers, M. (2002). Largest Religions in the United States. Washington, DC: The Pew Research Center. Retrieved from http://www.adherents.com/rel_USA.html#religions, July 24, 2007.

Linder, E. W. (Ed.) (2008). Yearbook of American and Canadian Churches. NY: National Council of Churches. Retrieved from http://www.electronicchurch.org. July 22, 2007.

O'Neil, D. (2008). Ethnicity and Race: An Introduction to the Nature of Social Group Differentiation and Inequality. San Marcos, CA: Palomar College. Retrieved from http://anthro.palomar.edu/ethnicity/Default.htm. February 18, 2008.

United States Census Bureau, Census 2000. Summary File 3, Tables P19, PCT13, and PCT14. Internet Release data: February 25, 2003. Retrieved from http://www.census.gov/population/cen2000/phc-t20/tab01.pdf, April 16, 2008.

United States Department of Education. (2007). No child left behind – High School Facts at a Glance. Retrieved from http://www.ed.gov/about/offices/list/ovae/pi/hs/hsfacts.html, October 18, 2007.

United States Department of Labor Statistics. (2008). Washington DC: United States Department of Labor. Retrieved from http://www.bls.gov/oes/current/oes_nat.htm#b00-0000, May 16, 2008.

United States Department of Health and Human Services. Fact Sheet – Your rights under Title VI of the Civil Rights Act. Retrieved from http://www.hhs.gov/ocr/generalinfo.html, July 15, 2007.

References

Abramson, H. J. (1980). Religion. In S. Thernstrom (Ed.), *Harvard encyclopedia of American ethnic groups*. Cambridge: Harvard University Press.

American Nurses' Association. (1993). *Proceedings of the invitational meeting, multicultural issues in the nursing workforce and workplace*. Washington, DC: Author.

Bohannan, P. (1992). *We, the alien—An introduction to cultural anthropology*. Prospect Heights, IL: Waveland Press.

Carroll, J. (2003). *Harley-Davidson: The living legend*. Edison, NJ: Edison Books.

Eck, D. L. (2001). *A new religious America: How a "Christian country" has become the world's most religious diverse nation*. San Francisco: Harper.

Estes, G., & Zitzow, D. (1980, November). *Heritage consistency as a consideration in counseling Native Americans*. Paper read at the National Indian Education Association Convention, Dallas, TX.

Fadiman A. (1997). *The spirit catches you and you fall down*. New York: Farrar, Straus, Giroux.

Fejos, P. (1959). Man, magic, and medicine. In L. Goldston (Ed.), *Medicine and anthropology*, New York: International University Press.

Giger, J. N., & Davidhizar, R. E. (1995). *Transcultural nursing assessment and intervention* (2nd ed.). St. Louis: Mosby-Year Book.

Hicks, R., & Hicks, K. (1999). *Boomers, Xers, and other strangers*. Wheaton, IL: Tyndale House.

Hunter, J. D. (1994). *Before the shooting begins—Searching for democracy in America's culture wars*. New York: Free Press.

LaFrombose, T., Coleman, L. K., & Gerton, J. (1993). Psychological impact of biculturalism: Evidence and theory. *Psychological Bulletin, 114*(3), 395.

Levin, J. (2001). *God, faith, and health*. New York: John Wiley & Sons.

Matsumoto, M. (1989). *The unspoken way*. Tokyo: Kodahsha International.

McLemore, S. D. (1980). *Racial and ethnic relations in America*. Boston: Allyn & Bacon.

Novak, M. (1973). How American are you if your grandparents came from Serbia in 1888? In S. Te Selle (Ed.), *The rediscovery of ethnicity: Its implications for culture and politics in America*. New York: Harper & Row.

Office of Minority Health. (2001). *National standards for culturally and linguistically appropriate services in health care*. Washington, DC: U.S. Department of Health and Human Services.

Senior, C. (1965). *The Puerto Ricans: Strangers then neighbors*. Chicago: Quadrangle Books.

Thernstrom, S. (Ed.). (1980). *Harvard encyclopedia of American ethnic groups*. Cambridge: Harvard University Press.

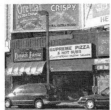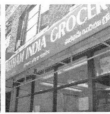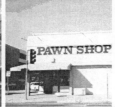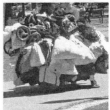

Chapter 2

Diversity

Demography is destiny.

—Hodgkinson (1986)

■ Objectives

1. Describe the total population characteristics of the United States as presented in Census 2000.
2. Compare the population characteristics of the United States from 1970 to 2000.
3. Discuss the changes in points of origin of recent and past immigrants.
4. Discuss the meanings of terms related to immigration, such as *citizen* and *refugee*.

This is now the 21st century and health care providers are entangled in the revolutionary consequences of enormous demographic, social, and cultural change. Many of these changes are playing a dramatic role both in the delivery of health care to patients, their families, and communities and in the workforce and environment in which the provider practices. The emerging majority—people of color—that constituted 19.7% of the population in 1990 in 2000 constituted 25% of the population; in 2005, the figure was 32% and is rapidly growing (U.S. Bureau of the Census, 1992, 2006). The comments and data presented in this chapter are designed to provide you with an image of the demographic features, derived from Census 2000, recent immigration, labor, and economic backgrounds of the American population.

In order to understand the profound changes that are taking place in the health care system, both in the delivery of services and in the profile of the people who are receiving and delivering services, we must look at the changes in the American population. The White majority is aging and shrinking; the Black, Hispanic, Asian, and American Indian populations are young and growing. It is imperative for those who deliver health care to be understanding of and sensitive to cultural differences and to the effect of the differences on a person's health and illness beliefs and practices and health care needs.

▓ Census 2000

Every census adapts to the decade in which it is conducted. One of the most important changes for Census 2000 was the revision of the questions that were asked regarding race and Hispanic origin. The federal government considers race and Hispanic origin to be two separate concepts and the questions on race and Hispanic origin were asked of all people living in the United States. The changes were developed to reflect the country's growing diversity. The respondents were given the option of selecting one or more race categories to indicate their racial identities. Given these changes, the Census 2000 data on race are not directly comparable with data from the 1990 Census or earlier censuses. However, for the purpose of comparison in this text, the data from the tables that factor in Hispanic origin and use the categories White and Black, alone, *non-Hispanic* will be used. Another factor that presents confusion is that people were free to define themselves as belonging to many groups. However, the overwhelming majority of the population reported one race.

In 1997 the Office of Management and Budget established federal guidelines to collect and present data on race and Hispanic origin. Census 2000 adhered to the guidelines, and established minimal categories as follows:

1. **White**—A person having origins in any of the original peoples of Europe, the Middle East, or North Africa. It includes people who indicate their race as "White" or report on entries such as Irish, German, Italian, or Arab.

2. **Black or African American**—A person having origins in any of the original black racial groups of Africa. It includes, for example, people who indicate their race as Black, African American, or Negro.

3. **American Indian and Alaska Native**—A person having origins in any of the original people of North and South America (including Central America) and who maintain tribal affiliation or community attachment.

4. **Asian**—A person having origins in any of the original people of the Far East, Southeast Asia, or the Indian subcontinent, including, for example, China, India, and the Philippine Islands.

5. **Native Hawaiian and Other Pacific Islander**—People who have origins in any of the original peoples of Hawaii, Guam, Samoa, or

other Pacific Islands or who provided a write-in response of a Pacific Islander group. This group has been clustered in the category of "other," as the percentages in the general population and age are small (Grieco & Cassidy, 2001, p. 2).

6. **Hispanic or Latino**—People who identify in categories such as Mexican, Puerto Rican, or Cuban, as well as those who indicate they are of other Spanish origin. Origin can be viewed as heritage, nationality group, lineage, or country of birth of the person or person's parents, or their ancestors before their arrival in the United States. People who identify their origin as Spanish can be of any race (Grieco & Cassidy, 2001, p. 2; Lew, 2000).

These terms of classification will be used throughout this chapter and the text. Since the census does not break down the population by gender, except male/female and by abled/disabled, this text will not include these variables in its discussions.

Total Population Characteristics

The 2000 census percentages are compared with the 1980 and 1990 census percentages. The figures demonstrate both the growth of the American population in general and the growth of people of color specifically. The changes are as follows:

1. In 1990, despite an accepted head count shortfall of 4.7 million people, the population count of the United States represented an increase of 22,167,670 people over the 1980 census and 19.8% of the population was comprised of people of color. Again, it may also be noted that 9.0% of the population claimed Hispanic or Spanish origin but could be of any race. Note that the European American majority had shrunk by about 3%, and there is an "emerging majority" of people of color.

2. In 2000, the population of the United States was counted as 281,421,906 (U.S. Bureau of the Census, 2006), which represented an increase of 32,712 (in thousands) from 1990, and 25% of the population was comprised of people of color. It may also be noted that 12.5% of the population claimed Hispanic or Latino origin but could be of any race.

3. During the fall of 2006, the population reached 300 million. In March 2008 the total population for the United States was 303,536,174. (U.S. Census Bureau, Retrieved March 1, 2008 from http://www.census.gov/index.html).

Age. The age classification is based on the age of the person in complete years as of April 1, 2000. The age was derived from the date of birth information requested on the census form. It is critical to note the following points regarding age in 2000:

▨ Twenty-six percent, or 72.3 million, of the U.S. population were under 18.

▓ Twenty-six percent, or 174.1 million, of the population were between 18 and 64.

▓ The percentage of the under-18-year-old populations was greater than the total population among Blacks, American Indians, and Hispanics.

▓ Twelve percent, or 35 million people, were age 65 or over.

▓ The percentage of the 65+ population was the greatest among White non-Hispanics (U.S. Bureau of the Census, 2001, p. 1 retrieved from http://www.census.gov).

American Indian, Aleut, and Eskimo Populations (Alone). The American Indian, Eskimo, and Aleut populations alone in the United States constituted 0.9% of the total population in 2000 and in 2005. The percentage of the population in 2000, under 18 was 33.9%; 18–24, 11%; 25–44, 30.9%; 45–64, 18.0%; and 65 and over, 5.6%. The median age of the population was 27.7 years in 2000.

Asian/Pacific Islander Population (Alone). Members of the Asian/Pacific Island communities made up 3.6% of the population in 2000 and 4.7% in 2005. The percentage of the population under 18 in 2000, was 24.1%; 18–24, 11.1%; 25–44, 36.0%; 45–64, 21%; and 65 and over, 7.8%. The median age of the Asian/Pacific Island population was 32.5 years in 2000.

Black Population (Alone). The Black population alone in the United States constituted 12.3% of the total population in 2000 and 12.8% in 2005. The percentage of the population under 18 in 2000, was 31.4%; 18–24, 11.0%; 25–44, 30.9%; 45–64, 18.6%; and 65 and over, 8.1%. The median age of the Black population was 30.0 years in 2000.

Hispanic Population (of Any Race). Hispanic Americans (of any race) made up 12.5% of the total population in 2000 and 14.4% in 2005. The percentage of the population under 18, was 35%; 18–24, 13.4%; 25–44, 33.0%; 45–64, 13.7%; and 65 and over, 4.9%. The median age of the Hispanic population was 25.8 years in 2000.

White Population (Alone). In 2000 the White population in the United States constituted 72.1% of the total population and 68% in 2005. The percentage of the population under 18 in 2000, was 23.5%; 18–24, 8.9%; 25–44, 29.6%; 45–64, 23.7%; 65 and over, 14.4%. The median age of the population was 38.6 years in 2000.

The U.S. Census Bureau produces estimates of the resident population for the United States on an annual basis. It revises the estimates time series each year as final input data become available. These postcensal estimates from April 1, 2000, through July 1, 2006, supersede all previous estimates produced since Census 2000. On March 30, 2007, the U.S. Census Bureau submitted to Congress the subjects it plans to address in the 2010 Census, which include gender, age, race, ethnicity, relationship, and whether you own or rent your home. It is estimated that the questions will take less than 10 minutes to complete. This indicates that the 2010 Census will be one of the shortest and easiest to complete since the nation's first census in 1790. There will also be a yearly American Community Survey, which will eliminate the need for a long-form questionnaire and will provide key socioeconomic and housing data about the nation's rapidly changing population.

Immigration

Immigrants and their descendants constitute most of the population of the United States, and Americans who are not themselves immigrants have ancestors who came to the United States from elsewhere. The only people considered native to this land are the American Indians, the Aleuts, and the Inuit (or Eskimos), for they migrated here thousands of years before the Europeans (Thernstrom, 1980, p. vii).

Immigrants come to the United States seeking religious and political freedom and economic opportunities. The life of the immigrant is fraught with difficulties—going from an "old" to a "new" way of life, learning a new language, and adapting to a new climate, new foods, and a new culture. Socialization of immigrants occurs in American public schools, and Americanization, according to Greeley (1978), is for some a process of "vast psychic repression," wherein one's language and other familiar trappings are shed. In part, the concept of the melting pot has been created in schools, where children learn English, reject family traditions, and attempt to take on the values of the dominant culture and "pass" as Americans (Novak, 1973). This difficult experience, as noted and described by Greeley and Novak in the 1970s, continues today.

A **citizen** of the United States is a native-born, foreign-born child of citizens, or a naturalized person who owes allegiance to the United States and who is entitled to its protection. "All persons born or naturalized in the United States, are citizens of the United States and of the state wherein they reside." A **refugee** is any person who is outside his or her country of nationality who is unable or unwilling to return to that country because of persecution or a well-founded fear of persecution. Persecution or the fear thereof must be based on the alien's race, religion, nationality, membership in a particular social group, or political opinion. People with no nationality must generally be outside their country of last habitual residence to qualify as a refugee. Refugees are subject to ceilings by geographic area set annually by the president in consultation with Congress and are eligible to adjust to lawful permanent resident status after 1 year of continuous presence in the United States. A permanent resident alien is an alien admitted to the United States as a lawful permanent resident. A "green card" provides official immigration status (lawful permanent residency) in the United States. Immigrants are now referred to as Legal Permanent Residents; however, the Immigration and Nationality Act (INA) broadly defines an immigrant as "any alien in the United States, except one legally admitted under specific nonimmigrant categories." An illegal alien, or undocumented person, who entered the United States without inspection, for example, would be strictly defined as an immigrant under the INA but is not a Legal Permanent Resident. Legal Permanent Residents are legally accorded the privilege of residing permanently in the United States. There are estimated (2007) to be 12 million undocumented people living in the United States.

In 2006, a total of 1,266,264 people became Legal Permanent Residents of the United States. The majority, 65%, already resided here. Among the LPRs Mexico, 14%; China, 7%; and the Philippines, 6% were the leading countries of birth (Jefferys, 2007, p. 1). In 1970, the highest percentage of people were from Europe, whereas in 2000 people from Mexico, China, and the Philippines were the highest in percentage.

In addition to the number of people entering the United States legally, there were 4.6 to 5.4 million undocumented immigrants residing here in 1996. It is extremely difficult to count the number of people who are hiding because they are not documented and estimated to be 12 million in 2007. It is widely recognized that the population is growing by about 275,000 people each year. California is the leading state of residence for undocumented people. Other states include Texas, New York, and Florida.

Explore 🌐 MediaLink

Go to the Companion Website at www.prenhall.com/spector for chapter-related review questions, case studies, and activities. Contents of the CulturalCare Guide and CulturalCare Museum can also be found on the Companion Website. Click on Chapter 2 to select the activities for this chapter.

■ Internet Sources

American Fact Finder Selected Characteristics of the Native and Foreign-Born Population, American Community Survey, 2005. (http://factfinder.census.gov/servlet/STTable?_bm=y&-geo_id=01000US&-) http://www.uscis.gov/ propub/ProPubVAP.jsp?dockey=2b289cf41dd6b70a61a078a9fbfbc379

Bernstein, R., Census Bureau, August 9, 2007, http://www.census.gov/Press-Release/www/releases/, August 9, 2007.

Grieco, E. and Cassidy, R. C. (2001). Overview of Race and Hispanic Origin. Census Brief. Washington, DC: Census Bureau. Retrieved from http://www.census.gov/prod/2001pubs/c2kbr01-1.pdf, July 25, 2007.

Hoefer, M., Rytina, N., and Campbell, C. (2007). Estimates of the Unauthorized Immigrant Population in the United States: January, 2006. Washington, DC: Department of Homeland Security. Retrieved March 1, 2008 from http://www.dhs.gov/ximgtn/statistics/publications/index.shtm

Jefferys, K. (2007). U.S. Legal Permanent Residents, 2006. Washington, DC: Department of Homeland Security. Retrieved March 1, 2008 from http://www.dhs.gov/ximgtn/statistics/publications/index.shtm

Lew, J. J. (2000). Guidance on Aggregation and Allocation of Data on Race for use in Civil Rights Monitoring and Enforcement. Washington, DC, Office of Man-

agement and Budget. Retrieved March 1, 2008 from http://www.whitehouse.
gov/omb/bulletins/b00-02.html

Nilsen, S. (2007). Poverty in America – Report to Congrssional Requesters. Washington, DC: United States Government Accountability Office. Retrieved July 21, 2007 from www.gao.gov/cgi-bin/getrpt

U.S. Census Bureau, "Annual Estimates of the Population by Sex, Age and Race for the United States: April 1, 2000 to July 1, 2005(NC-EST2005-04)"; published 10 May 2006; http://www.census.gov/popest/national/asrh/NCEST2005-asrh.html, http://www.uscis.gov/portal/site/uscis/menuitem.5af9bb95919 f35e66 f614176543f6dla/?vgnextoid=dcf5eldf53b2f010VgnVCM1000000ecd190a RCRD &vgnextchannel=d1fc9f9934741110VgnVCM1000000ecd190aRCRD

U.S. Census Bureau, Current Population Survey, 2006 Annual Social and Economic Supplement. *Last revised: August 29, 2006* http://pubdb3.census.gov/macro/032006/pov/new35_000.htm

United States Department of Homeland Security. (2007). United States History and Government Questions. Washington, DC: United States Citizenship and Immigration Services. Retrieved March 1, 2008 from http://www.dhs.gov/index.shtm

United States Department of Homeland Security. (2007). Press Release. Administration and Bipartisan Group of Senators Reach Bipartisan Agreement on Comprehensive Immigration Reform. Washington, DC: Department of Homeland Security. P. 1. Retrieved on March 1, 2008 from http://www.dhs.gov/xnews/releases/pr_1179511978687.shtm

United States Department of Homeland Security. (2007). United States History and Government Questions. Washington, DC: United States Citizenship and Immigration Services. Retrieved March 1, 2008 from http://www.uscis.gov/portal/site/uscis/menuitem.5af9bb95919f35e66f614176543f6d1a/?vgnextoid=12e596981298d010VgnVCM10000048f3d6a1RCRD&vgnextchannel=96719c7755cb9010VgnVCM10000045f3d6a1RCRD

References

Dalaku, J. (2001). *Poverty in the United States: 2000.* U.S. Census Current Population Reports Series P60–214. Wahington, DC: U.S. Government Printing Office.

Davis, F., & Furtado, C. (2002, July 22). INS to enforce change-of-address rule. *Boston Globe*, p. A2.

DeNavas-Walt, C., Proctor, B., & Lee, C. (2006). *Income, poverty, and health insurance coverage in the United States: 2005.* Washington, DC: U.S. Government Printing Office.

Greeley, A. (1978). *Why can't they be like us? America's white ethnic groups.* New York: E. P. Dutton.

Grieco, E. M., & Cassidy, R. C. (2001). *Overview of race and Hispanic origin.* Washington, DC: U.S. Census Bureau.

Hodgkinson, H. L. (1986, December). Reform? Higher education? Don't be absurd! *Higher Education*, 273.

Novak, M. (1973). How American are you if your grandparents came from Serbia in 1888? In S. Te Selle (Ed.), *The rediscovery of ethnicity: Its implications for culture and politics in America.* New York: Harper & Row.

Spector, M. (1979). Poverty: The barrier to health care. In R. E. Spector (Ed.), *Cultural diversity in health and illness* (pp. 141–162). New York: Appleton, Century & Crofts.

Thernstrom, S. (Ed.). (1980). *Harvard encyclopedia of American ethnic groups.* Cambridge: Harvard University Press.

U.S. Bureau of the Census. (1981, February 23). *1980 census population.* Press release CB81-32 and Supplementary report PC80-S1-1. Washington, DC: U.S. Government Printing Office.

U.S. Bureau of the Census. (1992, November). *1990 census of the population, general population characteristics United States.* Washington, DC: U.S. Government Printing Office.

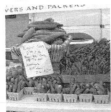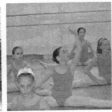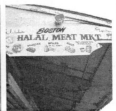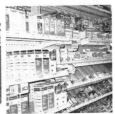

Chapter 3

Health and Illness

All things are connected. Whatever befalls the earth befalls the children of the earth.

—*Chief Seattle Suqwamish and Duwamish*

■ Objectives

1. Understand health and illness and the sociocultural and historical phenomena that affect them.
2. Reexamine and redefine the concepts of health and illness.
3. Understand the multiple relationships between health and illness.

There are countless images we can imagine to ponder comprehensive notions of health and illness. What do you do daily to maintain your health? What do you do when you experience a self-limiting ailment? How are ideas of health and illness reflected throughout the contemporary dominant culture in your home community? The community you work in? If you could pick four images relating to health and illness from your heritage, what would they be?

■ Health

The answers to the question "What is health?" are not as readily articulated as you might assume. One response may be a flawless recitation of the World Health Organization (WHO) definition of *health* as a "state of complete physical, mental, and social well being and not merely the absence of disease." This answer may be recited with great assurance—a challenge is neither expected nor welcomed but may evoke an intense dispute in which the assumed right answer is completely torn apart. Answers such as "homeostasis," "kinetic energy in balance," "optimal functioning," and "freedom from pain" are open to discussion. Experienced health care providers may be unable to give a comprehensive, acceptable answer to such a seemingly simple question. It is difficult to give a definition that makes sense without the use of some form of medical jargon. It is also challenging to define *health* in terms that a layperson can understand. (We lack skill in understanding "health" from the layperson's perspective.)

When you "Google" *health*, the response on the World Wide Web is well over 1.15 billion hits. One basic dictionary definition for the term is 1 : the condition of an organism or one of its parts in which it performs its vital functions normally or properly : the state of being sound in body or mind <dental *health*> <mental *health*>; *especially* : freedom from physical disease and pain <nursed him back to *health*> 2 : the condition of an organism with respect to the performance of its vital functions especially as evaluated subjectively or nonprofessionally <how is your *health* today>. Another one of the many classical definitions of *health* is in the *American Heritage Dictionary* (1976, p. 328):

> n. 1. The state of an organism with respect to functioning, disease, and abnormality at any given time. 2. The state of an organism functioning normally without disease or abnormality. 3. Optimal functioning with freedom from disease and abnormality. 4. Broadly, any state of optimal functioning, well being, or progress. 5. A wish for someone's good health, expressed as a toast.

As long ago as 1860, Florence Nightingale described health as "being well and using one's powers to the fullest extent." Murray and Zentner (1975) have classically defined *health* as "a purposeful, adaptive response, physically, mentally, emotionally, and socially, to internal and external stimuli in order to maintain stability and comfort." Rogers (1989) described health as "symbolic of wellness, a value term defined by culture or individual."

These definitions—varying in scope and context—are essentially those that the student practitioner, and educator within the health professions agree convey the meaning of *health*. The most widely used and recognized definition is that of WHO. Within the socialization process of the health care deliverer, the denotation of the word is that contained in the WHO definition. For other students, the meaning of the word *health* becomes clear through the educational experience.

▦ Illness

It is a paradox that the world of illness is the one that is most familiar to the providers of health care. It is in this world that the provider feels most comfortable and useful. Many questions about illness need to be answered:

- ▦ What determines illness?
- ▦ How do you know when you are ill?
- ▦ What provokes you to seek help from the health care system?
- ▦ At what point does self-treatment seem no longer possible?
- ▦ Where do you go for help? And to whom?

We tend to regard illness as the absence of health, yet we demonstrated in the preceding discussion that *health* is at best an elusive term that defies a specific definition. Let us look at the present issue more closely. Is illness the opposite of health? Is it a permanent condition or a transient condition? How do you know if you are ill?

When you "Google" *illness,* the response on the World Wide Web is well over 95.7 million hits. One basic dictionary definition for this term is an unhealthy condition of body or mind: SICKNESS (© 2005 by Merriam-Webster Incorporated). Another definition is found in the *American Heritage Dictionary* defines *illness* as "Sickness of body or mind. b. sickness. 2. obsolete. Evil; wickedness" (Davies, 1976, p. 351). A more contemporary definition of *illness* is "a highly personal state in which the person feels unhealthy or ill, may or may not be related to disease" (Kozier, Erb, Berman, & Burke 2000, p. 176). As with the word *health,* the word *illness* can be subjected to extensive analysis. What is illness? A generalized response, such as "abnormal functioning of a body's system or systems," evolves into more specific assessments of what we observe and believe to be wrong. Illness is a "sore throat," a "headache," or a "fever"—the last one determined not necessarily by the measurement on a thermometer but by a flushed face; a warm-to-hot feeling of the forehead, back, and abdomen; and overall malaise. The diagnosis of "intestinal obstruction" is described as pain in the stomach (abdomen), a greater pain than that caused by "gas," accompanied by severely upset stomach, nausea, vomiting, and marked constipation.

Essentially, we are being pulled back in the popular direction and encouraged to use lay terms. We initially resist this because we want to employ professional jargon. (Why use lay terms when our knowledge is so much greater?) It is crucial that we be called to task for using jargon. We must learn to be constantly conscious of the way in which the laity perceive illness and health care.

Another factor emerges as the word *illness* is stripped down to its barest essentials. Many of the characteristics attributed to health occur in illness, too. You may receive a rude awakening when you realize that a person perceived as healthy by clinical assessment may then—by a given set of symptoms—define him- or herself as ill (or vice versa). For example, in summertime, one may see a person with a red face and assume that she has a sunburn. The person may, in fact, have a fever. A person recently discharged from the hospital, pale and barely able to walk, may be judged ill. That individual may consider himself well, however, because he is much better than when he entered the hospital—now he is able to walk! Thus, perceptions are relative and, in this instance, the eyes of the beholder have been clouded by inadequate information. Unfortunately, at the provider's level of practice, we do not always ask the patient, "How do you view your state of health?" Rather, we determine the patient's state of health by objective and observational data.

As is the case with the concept of health, we learn in nursing or medical school how to determine what illness is and how people are expected to behave when they are ill. Once these terms are separated and examined, the models that health care providers have created tend to carry little weight. There is little agreement as to what, specifically, illness is, but we nonetheless have a high level of expectation as to what behavior should be demonstrated by both the patient and the provider when illness occurs. We discover that we have a vast amount of knowledge with respect to the acute illnesses and the services that ideally must be provided for the acutely ill person. When contradictions surface, however, it becomes apparent that our knowledge of the vast gray area is minimal—for example, whether someone is ill or becoming ill with what may later be an acute episode. Because of the ease with which we often identify cardinal symptoms, we find we are able to react to acute illness and may have negative attitudes toward those who do not seek help when the first symptom of an acute illness appears. The questions that then arise are "What is an acute illness, and how do we differentiate between it and some everyday indisposition that most people treat by themselves?" and "When do we draw the line and admit that the disorder is out of the realm of adequate self-treatment?"

These are certainly difficult questions to answer, especially when careful analysis shows that even the symptoms of an acute illness tend to vary from one person to another. In many acute illnesses, the symptoms are so severe that the person experiencing them has little choice but to seek immediate medical care. Such is the case with a severe myocardial infarction, but what about the person who experiences mild discomfort in the epigastric region? Such a symptom could lead the person to conclude he or she has "indigestion" and to self-medicate with baking soda, an antacid, milk, or Alka-Seltzer. A person who experiences mild pain in the left arm may delay seeking care, believing the pain will disappear. Obviously, this person may be as ill as the person who seeks help during the onset of symptoms but will, like most people, minimize these small aches because of not wanting to assume the sick role.

The Sick Role

The seminal work of Talcott Parsons (1966) helps explain the phenomenon of "the sick role." In our society, a person is expected to have the symptoms viewed as illness confirmed by a member of the health care profession. In other words, the sick role must first be legitimately conferred on this person by the keepers of this privilege. You cannot legitimize your own illness and have your own diagnosis accepted by society at large. There is a legitimate procedure for the definition and sanctioning of the adoption of the sick role and it is fundamental for both the social system and the sick individual. Thus, illness is not only a "condition" but also a social role. Parsons describes four main components of the sick role:

1. "The sick person is exempted from the performance of certain of his/her normal social obligations." An example is a student or worker who has a severe sore throat and decides that he or she does not want to go to classes or work. For this person to be exempted from the day's activities, he or she must have this symptom validated by someone in the health care system, a provider who is either a physician or a nurse practitioner. The claim of illness must be legitimized or socially defined and validated by a sanctioned provider of health care services.

2. "The sick person is also exempted from a certain type of responsibility for his/her own state." For example, an ill person cannot be expected to control the situation or be spontaneously cured. The student or worker with the sore throat is expected to seek help and then to follow the advice of the attending physician or nurse in promoting recovery. The student or worker is not responsible for recovery except in a peripheral sense.

3. "The legitimization of the sick role is, however, only partial." When you are sick, you are in an undesirable state and should recover and leave this state as rapidly as possible. The student's or worker's sore throat is acceptable only for a while. Beyond a reasonable amount of time—as determined by the physician or nurse, peers, and the faculty or supervisors—legitimate absence from the classroom or work setting can no longer be claimed.

4. "Being sick, except in the mildest of cases, is being in need of help." Bona fide help, as defined by the majority of American society and other Western countries, is the exclusive realm of the physician or nurse practitioner. A person seeking the help of the provider now not only bears the sick role but in addition takes on the role of patient. Patienthood carries with it a certain, prescribed set of responsibilities, some of which include compliance with a medical regimen, cooperation with the health care provider, and the following of orders without asking too many questions, all of which leads to the illness experience.

The Illness Experience

The experience of an illness is determined by what illness means to the sick person. Furthermore, *illness* refers to a specific status and role within a given society. Not only must illness be sanctioned by a physician for the sick person to assume the sick role, but it also must be sanctioned by the community or society structure of which the person is a member. Alksen and colleagues (n.d.) divide this experience into four stages, which are sufficiently general to apply to any society or culture.

The first stage, onset, is the time when the person experiences the first symptoms of a problem. This event can be slow and insidious or rapid and acute. When the onset is insidious, the patient may not be conscious of symptoms or may think that the discomfort will eventually go away. If, however, the onset is acute, the person is positive that illness has occurred and that immediate help must be sought. This stage is seen as the prelude to legitimization of illness. It is the time when the person with a sore throat in the preceding discussion may have experienced some fatigue, a raspy voice, or other vague symptoms.

In the second stage of the illness experience, diagnosis, the disease is identified or an effort is made to identify it. The person's role is now sanctioned, and the illness is socially recognized and identified. At this point, the health care providers make decisions pertaining to appropriate therapy. During the period of diagnosis, the person experiences another phenomenon: dealing with the unknown, which includes fearing what the diagnosis will be.

For many people, going through a medical workup is an unfamiliar experience. It is made doubly difficult because they are asked and expected to relate to strange people who are doing unfamiliar and often painful things to their bodies and minds. To the layperson, the environment of the hospital or the provider's office is both strange and unfamiliar, and it is natural to fear these qualities. Quite often, the ailing individual is faced with an unfamiliar diagnosis. Nonetheless, the person is expected to follow closely a prescribed treatment plan that usually is detailed by the health care providers but that, in all likelihood, may not accommodate a particular lifestyle. The situation is that of a horizontal-vertical relationship, the patient being figuratively and literally in the former position, the professional in the latter.

During the third stage, patient status, the person adjusts to the social aspects of being ill and gives in to the demands of his or her physical condition. The sick role becomes that of patienthood, and the person is expected to shift into this role as society determines it should be enacted. The person must make any necessary lifestyle alterations, become dependent on others in some circumstances for the basic needs of daily life, and adapt to the demands of the physical condition as well as to treatment limitations and expectations. The environment of the patient is highly structured. The boundaries of the patient's world are determined by the providers of the health care services, not by the patient. Herein lies the conflict.

Much has been written describing the environment of the hospital and the roles that people in such an institution play. As previously stated, the hospital is typically unfamiliar to the patient, who, nevertheless, is expected to conform to a predetermined set of rules and behaviors, many of which are unwritten and undefined for the patient—let alone by the patient.

The fourth stage—recovery—is generally characterized by the relinquishing of patient status and the assumption of prepatient roles and activities. There is often a change in the roles a person is able to play and the activities able to be performed once recovery takes place. Often, recovery is not complete. The person may be left with an undesirable or unexpected change in body image or in the ability to perform expected or routine activities. One example is a woman who enters the hospital with a small lump in her breast and who, after a surgery, returns home with only one breast. Another example is that of a man who is a laborer and enters the hospital with a backache and returns home after a laminectomy. When he returns to work, he cannot resume his job as a loader. Obviously, an entire lifestyle must be altered to accommodate such newly imposed changes.

From the viewpoint of the provider, this person has recovered. His or her body no longer has the symptoms of the acute illness that made surgical treatment necessary. In the eyes of the former patient, illness persists because of the inability to perform as in the past. So many changes have been wrought that it should come as no surprise if the person seems perplexed and uncooperative. Here, too, there is certainly conflict between society's expectations and the person's expectation. Society releases the person from the sick role at a time when, subjectively, the person may not be ready to relinquish it.

Internet Sources

Office of Disease Prevention and Health Promotion. (2005). Healthy People 2010 Rockville, MD: U.S. Department of Health and Human Service. Retrieved from http://www.healthypeople.gov/, June 22, 2007.

References

Alksen, L., Wellin, E., Suchman, E., et al. (n.d.). *A conceptual framework for the analysis of cultural variations in the behavior of the ill.* Unpublished report (p. 2). New York: New York City Department of Health.

Davies, P. (Ed.). (1976). *The American heritage dictionary of the English language.* New York: Dell.

Kozier, B., Erb, G., Berman, A. J., & Burke, K. (2000). *Fundamentals of nursing concepts, process, and practice.* Upper Saddle River, NJ: Prentice Hall Health.

Mechanic, D. (1968). *Medical sociology* (p. 80). New York: Free Press of Glencoe.

Murray, R., & Zentner, J. (1975). *Nursing concepts for health promotion.* Englewood Cliffs, NJ: Prentice Hall.

National Center for Health Statistics [NCHS]. (2007). *Health United States 2007.* Hyattsville, MD: Author.

Nightingale, F. (1860, 1946). (A fascimile of the first edition published by D. Appleton and Co.). *Notes on nursing—What it is, what it is not.* New York: Appleton-Century.

Parsons, T. (1966). Illness and the role of the physician: A sociological perspective. In W. R. Scott & E. H. Volkart (Eds.), *Medical care: Readings in the sociology of medical institutions* (p. 275). New York: John Wiley & Sons.

Rogers, M. (1989). Nursing: A science of unitary human beings. In Riehl-Sisca, J. (Ed.), *Conceptual models for nursing practice* (3rd ed., pp. 181–188). Norwalk, CT: Appleton & Lange.

Rosenstock, I. M. (1966, July). Why people use health services. *Millbank Memorial Fund Quarterly, 44*(3), 94–127.

Suchman, E. A. (1965, fall). Stages of illness and medical care. *Journal of Health and Human Behavior, 6*(3), 114.

Unit

II

HEALTH
Domains

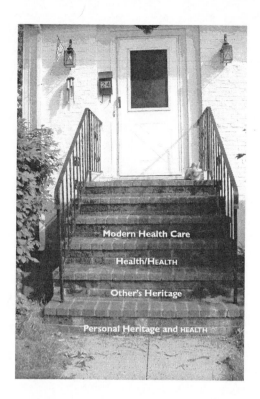

Unit II develops the "plot" of this book by providing background material for the central themes discussed in this text. Imagine climbing the stairs in the opening figure and this unit will bring you to the fifth step.

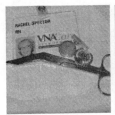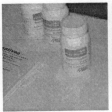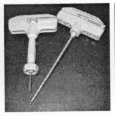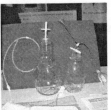

Chapter 4

Health Care Delivery and Issues

■ Objectives

1. Discuss the professional socialization of nurses, physicians, and other members of the health care delivery system.
2. Describe the "culture" of the health care providers.
3. Discuss the costs of health care both as a national issue and as an issue in the area you reside.
4. Recognize the interrelationships and trends of sociocultural, public health, and medical events that have produced the crises in today's modern health care system.
5. Chart the "Amazing Maze of Health Care" and give examples of your personal and professional experience.
6. Describe barriers to health care.

The chapter-opening images depict symbols related to the modern health care delivery culture and objects used to maintain or restore overall health. The first image portrays selected cultural objects—a nametag, bandage scissors, my school of nursing pin, and a volunteer pin from the American Red Cross. The second image symbolizes medications—whether given to maintain health (for example, vitamins or calcium) or to treat ailments from cardiovascular diseases to mental illnesses, one thing is certain—the costs are usually exorbitant. The third and fourth images depict thoracotomy instruments—the trochanters and underwater chest tube drainage bottles represent the tremendous amount of medical equipment now available that is disposable and the constantly rising costs of all aspects of health care. In fact, as will be discussed in this chapter, it has been frequently demonstrated that the high cost of health care is not proof of high quality (Abelson, 2007, p. A-1) What are the unique symbols of your profession within the overall culture of modern health care? What objects would you choose to represent your experiences of modern health care delivery?

The health care system of this nation has been in crisis, and the visionary words and observations of Dr. John Knowles in 1970 ring true today:

> American medicine, the pride of the nation for many years, stands on the brink of chaos. Our medical practitioners have their great moments of drama and triumph. But, much of U.S. medical care, particularly the everyday business of preventing and treating illness, is inferior in quality, wastefully dispensed, and inequitably financed.

What is it about our health care system and the people who practice within it that generated and continue to generate these comments? This chapter presents an overview of the issues inherent in the acculturation of health care providers and the health care delivery system in the United States. It begins by discussing the norms of the health care provider "cultures" and then examines many of the salient issues regarding the health care system in general.

▨ The Health Care Provider's Culture

The providers of health care—nurses; physicians; social workers; dietitians; physical, occupational, respiratory, and speech therapists; laboratory and departmental professionals—are socialized into the culture of their profession. Professional socialization teaches the student a set of beliefs, practices, habits, likes, dislikes, norms, and rituals. Each of the professional disciplines has its own language and objects, rituals, garments, and myths, which become an inherent part of the scope of students' education, socialization, and practice. The providers view time in their own ways and they believe that their view of a health and illness situation and subsequent interventions are the only possible answers to the complex questions surrounding a health-related event. This newly learned information regarding health and illness differs in varying degrees from that of the individual's heritage. As students become more and more immersed and knowledgeable in the scientific and technological domains, they usually move further and further from their past belief systems and, indeed, futher from the population at large in terms of its understanding and beliefs regarding health/HEALTH and illness/ILLNESS. Just as it is not unusual to hear providers say, "Etoh, bid, tid, im, iv," and so forth, it is not uncommon to hear patients say things such as "I have no idea what the nurses and doctors are saying!" "They speak a foreign language!" "What they are doing is so strange to me." In addition, there exists an underlying cultural norm among health care providers that "all must be done to save a patient, regardless of the patient's and family's wishes" and regardless of the financial consequences to the patient and family, to the health care system, or to society in general. A consequence of this philosophy has been the rise of iatrogenic health problems and the escalation of out-of-control health care costs.

As a result, health care providers can be viewed as an alien or foreign culture or ethnic group. They have a social and cultural system; they experience "ethnicity" in the way they perceive themselves in relation to the health care consumer and often each other. Even if they deny the reality of the situation, health care providers must understand that they are ethnocentric. Not only are they ethnocentric, but also many of them are xenophobic. To appreciate this critical issue, consider the following. A principal reason for the difficulty experienced between the health care provider and the consumer is that health care providers, in general, adhere rigidly to the modern allopathic, or Western, system of health care delivery. (These terms may be used interchangeably to describe health care.) With few exceptions, they do not publicly sanction any methods of protection or healing other than scientifically proved ones. They ordinarily fail to recognize or use any sources of medication other than those that have been deemed effective by scientific means. The only types of healers that are sanctioned are those that have been educated, licensed, and certified according to the requirements of this culture.

What happens, then, when people of one belief system encounter people who have other beliefs regarding health and illness (either in protection or in treatment)? Is the provider able to meet the needs as perceived and defined by the patient? More often than not, a wall of misunderstanding arises between the two. At this point, a breakdown in communications occurs, and the consumer ends up at a disadvantage.

Providers think that they comprehend all facets of health and illness and may frequently take a xenophobic view to HEALTH and ILLNESS and traditional HEALERS. Although in training and education health care providers have a significant advantage over the consumer-patient, it is entirely appropriate for them to explore other ideas regarding health/HEALTH and illness/ILLNESS and to adjust their approach to coincide with the needs of the specific patient. Health care providers have tried to force Western medicine on one and all, regardless of results.

The following list outlines the more obvious aspects of the health care provider's culture. In connection with later chapters, it can be referred to as a framework for comparing various other ethnic and cultural beliefs and practices.

1. Beliefs
   a. Standardized definitions of *health* and *illness*
   b. The omnipotence of technology
2. Practices
   a. The maintenance of health and the protection of health or prevention of disease through such mechanisms as the avoidance of stress and the use of immunizations
   b. Annual physical examinations and diagnostic procedures, such as Pap smears, mammographies, and colonoscopies.

3. Habits
   a. Charting
   b. The constant use of jargon
   c. The use of a systematic approach and problem-solving methodology
4. Likes
   a. Promptness
   b. Neatness and organization
   c. Compliance
5. Dislikes
   a. Tardiness
   b. Disorderliness and disorganization
6. Customs
   a. Professional deference and adherence to the pecking order found in autocratic and bureaucratic systems
   b. Hand washing
   c. The use of certain procedures attending birth and death
7. The expectation of recovery no matter the cost or consequences of therapy

As noted, inherent in the socialization into the health care professions, nursing, medicine, social work, and the various therapies, there are countless cultural traits that are passed on both verbally and nonverbally. The doors in Figure 4–1 illustrate the closed aspects of the entire health care system.

We are now living in the 21st century, the third millennium; the problems of health care delivery have grown exponentially, and solutions are more elusive than ever. Doctors in the United States administer the world's most expensive medical (illness) care system. The costs of U.S. health care soared from $4 billion in 1940 to the 2000 figure of 1.4 trillion and to 1.9 trillion in 2005 (NCHS, 2007, p. 374). Health care is an enterprise that exceeds all the goods and services produced by half the states in the country.

Figure 4-1   The doors to a surgical suite. In contrast to the transparent door found in the Preface, this door is symbolic of the closed culture of modern health care delivery. Few people outside of this system understand the intricacies of the cultures of the health care providers and the system within which they practice.

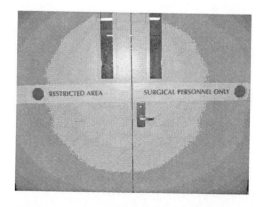

A recently published study by the Kaiser Family Foundation points out that:

▩ Health care costs have grown on average 2.5 percentage points faster than U.S. gross domestic product since 1970.

▩ Almost half of health care spending is used to treat just 5 percent of the population.

▩ Prescription drug spending is 10 percent of total health spending, but contributes to 14 percent of the growth in spending (Henry J. Kaiser Family Foundation, 2007, p.1).

Health Care Costs

The health care system is both a source of national pride—if one has an expensive and adequate health insurance package or the money, it certainly is possible to get the finest medical/technological care in the world—and a source of deep embarrassment—those who are poor or uninsured may be wanting for care. In fact, an estimated 16.4% of Americans under 65 years of age do not have health insurance (NCHS, 2006, p. 400). Other notable trends include

▩ The number and percentage of people covered by employment-based health insurance declined in 2004, from 66.7% in 2000 to 63.5% in 2004 (NCHS, 2006, p. 396).

▩ The percentage of uninsured children under 18 years dropped from 12.6% in 2000 to 9.2% in 2004 (NCHS, 2006, p. 400); however, children in low-income families remained more likely than children in higher-income families to lack coverage (NCHS, 2006, p. 12).

▩ In 2004, 30% of young adults 18–24 years of age were uninsured at a point in time (NCHS, 2006, p. 12).

▩ Of the people under 65 years old who were without health insurance in 2004,
  • 17.9% were male
  • 23.5% were between the ages of 18 and 44
  • 34.4% were Hispanic (NCHS, 2006, p. 400)

In addition

▩ Many people under 65 years of age, particularly those with a low family income, do not have consistent health insurance.

▩ The average percentage of the population with no health insurance coverage ranged from less than 10% in Minnesota, Hawaii, and Iowa to 25% in Texas.

▩ About one-half of the uninsured population were non-Hispanic white persons with the other half being people of other races and ethnicities (NCHS, 2007, p. 14).

Almost 50% of the American public say they are very worried about having to pay more for their health care or health insurance, while 42% report they are very worried about not being able to afford health care services. Three questions then present themselves:

1. Is health care in America better than in any other place on Earth?
2. What really are the costs of health care?
3. Why is health care so expensive?

Despite the high expenditures for health care, we were not healthier in 2004 than people from other nations. Infant mortality rate is the figure used as a standard for measuring the overall health of a nation. Infant mortality rates in the United States have been steadily declining since 1960 and the national average stands at 6.8 deaths per 1,000 births, yet, some southern states are experiencing a rise in their infant mortality rates. For example, Mississippi has had the biggest increase in the number of babies dying in their first year of life, and between 2004 and 2005 the rate was 11.4 deaths per 1,000 births. In fact, 26 other nations had lower infant mortality rates than the United States.

The sources for paying for care in 1960 were primarily personal, out of pocket or private insurance; Medicare and Medicaid did not yet exist—they were "born" in 1965. It is obvious that they now make over 50% of health care expenditures possible—coverage shifted from the private sector to the public sector and is presently shifting back to the private sector. Technology has exploded, the costs of health care have soared, and many of the health care–related programs are seen as "entitlements." The costs of services are blindly covered and quite often it is impossible for a patient to get an itemized bill, yet, when people get them, they are astonished at the costs but state, "My insurance covers it and it costs me nothing." However, for more and more people the costs of heath care have become so high that their health insurance companies either disallow desired procedures or stop payments after a certain amount is reached. Families are left bankrupt in many instances or finding it necessary to choose between care or financial insolvency.

The following examples illustrate the situation. As you read these examples, think about the events that may have occurred in the settings in which you deliver or receive care:

- Medication problems. In addition to the chronic, ongoing situation of medication errors, countless health care providers are "on the take and complicit with big business," gravely endangering our health and adding to the high costs of pharmaceuticals and other medical supplies (Kassirer, 2005, pp. 42–50).
- Quality of care errors. For example, one in three hospitals nationwide fail to ask patients on admission to list the medications they are taking (Kowalczyk, 2007b, p. A-1).
- Emergency room (department) errors. Patients may not be tended to in an appropriate manner. In fact, the wait in the emergency room can be as long as 8 hours and many patients may be left to wait in hallways (Kowalczyk, 2007a, p. A-1). In addition, the deeply embedded attitudes about race may influence the care doctors administer to African American patients in the emergency room (Smith, 2007, p. A-1).

▓ Dumping. Recently, patients have been dumped by physicians, insurance plans, and/or exisiting health maintenance organizations. It is extremely difficult and frustrating to find new providers that are covered by an insurance company's network. This phenomena is particularly difficult for people over 65 and on Medicare.

▓ Discredited medications, such as Avandia, used to treat diabetes. Patients given Avandia were found to have a 43% greater chance of developing a heart attack (Saul, 2007, p. A6).

▓ Diagnoses of bipolar disease in children. There has been a backlash on the frequent diagnosis of this disease (Allen, 2007, p. A-1), and the psychiatrists who have been ordering drugs, such as Risperdal, for children are being scrutinized (Harris, Carey, & Roberts, 2007, p. A1).

▓ False claims for OxyContin. The maker of OxyContin has been found guilty of making false claims of effects and misleading doctors about the chances of abuse of this drug and must pay a $600 million fine (Meier, 2007, p. A1).

The third question—"Why is it that health care is so expensive?"—may be answered by exploring the trends in the development of the health care system, but factored into this analysis is also the increase in the population; the desire by health care providers, researchers, and vendors to cure all diseases; and the public's expectation that all illnesses can be cured.

▓ Trends in Development of the Health Care System

During the days of the early colonists, our health care system was a system of superstition and faith. It has evolved into a system predicated on a strong belief in science; the epidemiological model of disease; highly developed technology; and strong values of individuality, competition, and free enterprise. Two major forces—free enterprise and sciences—have largely shaped the problems we now face. Health problems have evolved from the epidemics of 1850 to the chronic diseases of today, notwithstanding the resurgence of tuberculosis and the AIDS epidemic. In 1850, health care technology was virtually nonexistent; today, it dominates the delivery of health care. We now take for granted such dramatic procedures as kidney, heart, and liver transplants. New technologies and biomedical milestones are materializing daily (Torrens, 1988, pp. 3–31). However, the consequences of these events are also rising daily in terms of extraordinary costs and countless practice issues and errors, discussed earlier.

Social organizations and peer review bodies to control the use of technology did not exist in 1850; today they proliferate, and the federal government is expected to play a dominant role. The belief that health care is a right for all Americans is still a prominent philosophy, yet the fulfillment of that right is still in question. The trends, begun in the 1980s and early 1990s, such as the cutbacks in federal funding for health services and the attempt to turn the clock back on social programs have led to a diminished and denigrated role for the government in people's health. On the other hand, the events of September 11,

2001, have pointed out the consequences of these cuts and the enormous and compelling need to boost public health and national security efforts.

There is growing and grave concern about the realization of this basic human right of health and health care. Mounting social problems, such as toxic waste, homelessness, and millions of people without health insurance, confound the situation. These factors all affect the delivery of health care. The problems of acquiring and using the health care system are legendary and ongoing.

The year 1960 is the benchmark being used to compare health care costs and significant events. A brief overview of these landmark events follows. These events have contributed to what we see today as the health care "nightmare." We are in a situation where health care delivery has become less and less personal and more and more technological in many health care settings. The barriers to health care are increasing and, as evidenced earlier, more and more people are unable to obtain health care, in spite of having health insurance. The events depicted that have occurred in the health care system, whether within the public health or medical sector, have happened within the context of the longer societal framework. The public sector events include those related to the collective responsibility for the health of large populations in many dimensions—prevention, surveillance, disease control, and so forth—and those events, positive and negative, that affect large population cohorts. The medical events are those that include the development of diagnostic and/or therapeutic methods that are problem-specific and affect limited numbers of people. The public health events include government laws and policies that were designed initially to increase the scope of the health care system and later to control medical costs.

This information is further embedded in the key health system issues of the century and the start of this decade, the key health problems, and selected key health strategies of the time. The key issues are professionalization, infrastructure building, improved access, cost control, market forces, and the reinvention of government. The key health problems are reemerging infectious disease, chronic diseases, and the modern care changes. Key health strategies include maternal and infant health, antibiotics, screen and treat, and managed care.

At the turn of the 20th century, 1900–1930, efforts were underway to identify medicine as a profession and to eradicate all philosophies of care that were not under the umbrella of the Flexner definition of a profession. Agents such as quinine for malaria and the diphtheria antitoxin for immunization were discovered, and the use of radium to treat cancer began.

Infectious diseases, including pneumonia and influenza, were pandemic. The main health strategy was maternal and child health, given the large numbers of new immigrants. In 1929, third-party payment for health care began with the creation of Blue Cross and Blue Shield.

Between 1930 and 1960, the health care system issue was infrastructure building. The passage of the Hill-Burton Act in 1946 provided funding for the building of hospitals and other health care resources. The system was on a roll—the development of today's extraordinarily costly tests and treatments began, and the settings for their use were built. The development of vaccines and antibiotics paved the way to a decrease in the occurrence of communicable disease, and a false sense of freedom from illness began to develop. At the same time, it began to become obvious that, for many, access to health care was becoming more and more difficult.

In 1965, President Lyndon B. Johnson's War on Poverty became the focal point of social and health policy and, among other laws, Medicare and Medicaid came into being. The Health Professionals Education Assistance Act was passed, which led to the proliferation of medical nursing and other allied health programs. In 1967, the first heart transplant was performed by Dr. Christiaan Barnard in South Africa, and a whole new focus on science and technology was born. Today, transplants have become nearly ordinary events, and an entitlement philosophy is applied to receiving them.

The 1960s were an explosive time—there were too many assassinations, too many riots—yet strides were made in the struggle for civil rights. The war in Vietnam was a nightly television event until the truce in 1975. The 1970s, 1980s, and 1990s all had their share of strife and progress. Progress in health care was accompanied by the escalation of costs and the limiting of comprehensive care. The cases of HIV/AIDS continue to increase, and the threat of anthrax and other forms of bioterrorism are present in the minds of most people. In addition, the 1960s were a decade of profound change in the delivery of health care, public health, and available methods of treating health problems and funding new resources. Selected highlights include the

- Development of the vaccines for polio and rubella (1961 and 1963)
- Development of the methods for external cardiac pacing (1961)
- Development of liver transplant method (1963) and first human heart transplanted (1967)
- Surgeon General's Report on Smoking (1964)
- War on Poverty Medicare/Medicaid passed (1965)

The 1970s brought even greater strides in medical technology and public health:

- Professional Standards Review Organization established, Clean Water Act passed, and the Tuskegee experiment[1] ended (1972)
- Comprehensive Health Planning; "Certificate of Need" (1974)
- HBV—the hepatitis vaccine was developed (1978)
- First test tube baby born (1978)
- Biotechnical Explosion (1979)
- Cyclosporine developed (1979)

At the end of the 1970s, efforts were developed to "control" the costs of health care, yet the seductiveness of the "advances" in technology actually began the out-of-control escalation of the rise of health care costs. The following are ex-

---

[1]The Tuskegee syphilis experiment began in 1932.

amples of events in the 1980s that further fed the rising costs of health care and the emerging expectation of people to be entitled to better and better levels of technological diagnosis and illness care that would provide longer life expectancies:

- Nuclear magnetic resonance introduced (1980)
- The beginning of the HIV/AIDS epidemic and the HIV virus isolated at the Institute Pasteur, Paris (1981)
- Monoclonal antibodies (1984)
- Retroviral oncogenes (1985)

The 1990s to the present time have presented even greater challenges to the availability and affordability of health care. In 1993 and 1994, President and Mrs. Clinton made an extraordinary effort to study our complex health care system and sought ways to reform it. That effort did not materialize, and the present political energy has shifted from health care reform to welfare reform and the saving of Social Security and Medicare. The nation's 76 million baby boomers will soon be able to retire, which will necessitate large payouts from Social Security and Medicare, but it is unknown how many workers there will be to contribute to the system. The size of the shortfall depends on the changes in longevity, the birth rate, and immigration rates (Zitner, 1999). Efforts such as managed care (Saltus, 1999) and the discounting of payments for medications for the elderly were short-term and controversial approaches to managing funds. These efforts, too, have not succeeded.

Meanwhile, the costs of health care continue to soar, causing some hospitals to downsize their nursing staff in an effort to reduce costs. Ultimately, it was believed that the Clinton plan would create a few giant insurers, and health maintenance organizations (HMOs) would dominate the market; most people would be forced into low-cost plans, doctors would be employed by the insurers or HMOs, hospitals would be controlled by insurers and HMOs, care would be multitiered, the bureaucracy would increase, costs would not be contained, and financing would be regressive. The overall goal of health care reform was to make health care accessible, comprehensive, and affordable—a right and not a privilege of all residents of the United States. However, technology is advancing and our use of it is increasing, and we continue to spend vast sums on the care of patients in the last year of life while delivering less and less preventive care. In addition, the costs of for-profit care continue to explode, and the dominant force in managed care is the for-profit HMO.

The following are examples of health care events in the 1990s and early 2000:

- Human Genome Project (1992)
- Assisted suicide; Dr. J. Kevorkian (1996)
- Hantavirus pulmonary syndrome (1993)
- Septuplets born and survive (1997)

- Octuplets born; seven survive (1998)
- Stem cell cloning (1998)
- Biologics and follow-on biologics (2004)

With the catastrophe of September 11, 2001, the need to immunize people for smallpox and countless other public health issues emerged, as did the need for emergency preparedness.

Biologics are complex medicines that are manufactured with the use of living organisms. The increasing use of biologics and new follow-on biologics are the cutting edge of pharmaceutical therapies. The biogeneric market is about $2 billion. The Biotechnology Industry Organization (BIO) has stated that "the safety and effectiveness of a chemical drug can be established by the specification of its active ingredient, but the safety and effectiveness of a biotech product is determined by the manner in which it is made" (Samalonis, 2004). In other words, the consequences of this pioneering medicine will be expensive iatrogenic problems.

Grave concern is being expressed regarding the high costs of health care, the fact that between 16.1% and 17.5% of the population under 65 has no health insurance, that the costs of durable medical supplies and medications continue to rise, and so on. On one hand, we are seeking to ever expand therapeutic miracles; on the other hand, there is shock and dismay at the ever-increasing costs of health care.

▓ Pathways to Health Services

When a health problem occurs, there is an established system whereby health care services are obtained. The classical theoretical work that was developed in the mid-1960s and the 1970s continues to establish a viable framework for describing sources of patient problems. Suchman (1965) contends that the family is usually the first resource. It is in the domain of the family that the person seeks validation that what he or she is experiencing is indeed an illness. Once the belief is validated, health care outside of the home is sought. It is not unusual for a family to be receiving care from many different providers, with limited or no communication among the attending caregivers. Problems and complications erupt when a provider is not aware that other providers are caring for a patient. Let us not forget that, in rural and remote areas, comprehensive health care is difficult to obtain. For patients who are forced to use the clinics of a hospital, there is certainly no continuity of care because intern and resident physicians come and go each year. This is known as the level of first contact, or the entrance into the health care system.

The second level of care, if needed, is found at the specialist's level: in clinics, private practice, or hospitals. Obstetricians, gynecologists, surgeons, neurologists, and other specialists make up a large percentage of those who practice in medicine. Recently, hospitalists have been added.

The third level of care is delivered within hospitals that provide inpatient care and services. Care is determined by need, whether long-term (as in a psychiatric setting or rehabilitation institute) or short-term (as in the acute care setting and community hospitals).

An in-depth discussion of the different kinds of hospitals—voluntary or profit-making and nonprofit institutions—is more appropriate to a book dealing solely with the delivery of health care (see the Bibliography at the end of this book). In our present context, the issue is "what does the patient know about such settings, and what kind of care can he or she expect to receive?"

To many students, the health care delivery problems of a given hospital unit are far removed from the scope of practice they know from nursing school and from what they ordinarily see in a work setting (unless they choose to work in a city or county public hospital). Many students assume that the care they observe and deliver in a suburban or community private hospital is the universal norm. This is a fundamental error in experience and understanding, which can be corrected if students are assigned to visit first the emergency room of a city hospital and then the emergency room of a suburban hospital in order to compare the two milieus. Unless students visit each setting, they fail to gain an appreciation of the major differences—how vastly such facilities differ in the scope of patients' treatment. Students typically report that, in the suburban emergency room, the patients are called by name, their families wait with them, and every

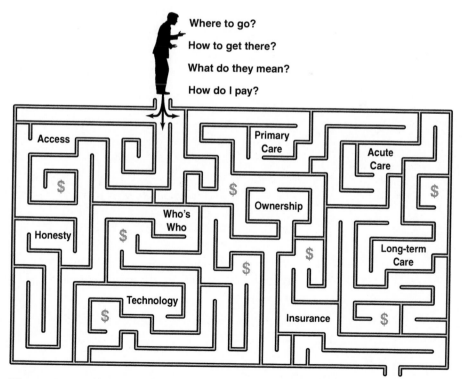

Figure 4-2 Navigating the amazing maze of health care.

effort is made to hasten their visit. The contrast with people in urban emergency rooms—who have waited for extended periods of time, are sometimes not addressed by name, and are not allowed to have family members come with them while they are examined—is astounding. The noise and confusion are also factors that confront and dismay students when they are exposed to big-city emergency rooms.

Figure 4–2 illustrates the maze of health care and the variety of obstacles a patient must deal with in attempting to navigate this complex system. Indeed, the patient not only needs to navigate an internal system of a given hospital but also needs to understand all the types of care available. Just to complicate matters more deeply, many people are given information that contradicts itself—as with the diagnosis and treatment of breast cancer or the use of estrogen replacement therapy—and then the patient is asked to make the choices.

■ Barriers to Health Care

There are countless factors, or barriers, in addition to financial that thwart a person's or family's ability to use the health care system to its greatest potential. The following are some examples:

Access	A person is unable to enter into the system because he or she lacks money, health insurance, or the ability to get to a center where health care is delivered. Another access factor is that primary care physicians are leaving their practices, either to retire or to limit the scope of their practices to "concierge" services.
Age	The person is too young or too old to enter into the system and is unaware of ways to overcome this.
Class	A person may be from a class that is not part of the dominant culture, limiting their ability to determine the need for health care and to understand the subtleties involved in making health care system choices.
Education	A person may not know how to read and write English and may not read and write in his or her native tongue.
Gender	Existing services may be limited to a specific gender or the person may be unwilling or unable to access a system that does not deliver gender-specific care.

(continued)

Geography	A person may not reside near a health care facility, and the costs of traveling to a facility may be unaffordable.
Homelessness	A person may be homeless in a place where health care is not provided to people who are homeless and the person does not know the ways to access the system.
Insurance	A person may not have health insurance or it may be inadequate to cover the scope of the person's needs.
Language	A person may not speak or understand English and adequate interpreter services may not be available.
Manners	A person's manners or expectations of the provider's manners may not be congruent.
Philosophy	The philosophy of an institution may not be congruent with a person's religious or personal philosophy.
Prejudice	The person seeking health care may sense the prejudice that the providers and institution exhibit.
Race	There may be residuals of racial prejudice as part of the institution's philosophy.
Racism	The institution may have specific barriers in place to not treat people from other races than the race of the owners of the facility.
Religion	A patient may not desire to be treated in an institution that is not derived from his or her religious background and there may be manifest prejudice on both sides—patient and institution.
SES (socio economic status)	The 2 extremes of socioeconomic status, poverty or great wealth, poverty can limit access to care and wealth may prevent people from seeking care in institutions where they prefer to not go because of the patient population served there.
Technology	A person may not be able to afford or want the plethora of diagnostic tests and therapies offered to him or her.
Transportation	There may be no public transportation available from where the patient resides to the institution.

In this chapter, we have explored, in a very limited way, the culture and characteristics inherent in the socialization into the health care professions; many of the issues surrounding the American health care delivery system by examining the history and trends that led to its present character; the experiences a person may have in attempting to obtain care; and how medicine is now an institution of social control.

The struggles continue as we attempt to find a balance between the high technology of the 21st century and primary preventive care and a strong public health care system. There must also be a balance between the forces of modern medical care and CULTURALCARE.

Explore ⊕ MediaLink

Go to the Companion Website at www.prenhall.com/spector for chapter-related review questions, case studies, and activities. Contents of the CulturalCare Guide and CulturalCare Museum can also be found on the Companion Website. Click on Chapter 7 to select the activities for this chapter.

▓ Internet Sources

Agency for Health Care—Florida. (2003). FloridaHealthFinder.gov. State of Florida Author. Retrieved July 2, 2007 from http://www.floridahealthfinder.gov/about-ahca/about-ahca.shtml

California Health Care Foundation. (2006). California Employer Health Benefits Survey, 2006. Oakland, CA: California HealthCare Foundation, Retrieved from http://www.chcf.org/topics/healthinsurance/index.cfm, March 2, 2008.

Henry J. Kaiser Family Foundation. (2005). The USA Today/Kaiser Family Foundation/Harvard School of Public Health—Health Care Costs Survey. Menlo Park, CA: Author. pub. #7371. Retrieved March 2, 2008 from http://www.kff.org/

Henry J. Kaiser Family Foundation (2007). Key Information on Health Care Costs and Their Impact. Menlo Park, CA: Author. Retrieved March 2, 2008 from http://www.kff.org/.

Samalonis, L.B. (2004). Follow-on biologies: The next frontier. Retrieved June 27, 2007 from http://www.drugtopics.com/drugtopics/article/articleDetail.jsp?id=115886

National Coalition on Health Care. (2008). Health Insurance Cost. Washington, DC: Author. Retrieved on March 2, 2008 from http://www.nchc.org/facts/cost.shtml

▓ References

Abelson, R. (2007, June 14). In health care, cost isn't proof of high quality. *New York Times*, p. A-1.

Allen, S. (2007, May 20). Backlash on bipolar diagnoses in children, *Boston Globe*, p. A-1.

Dembner, A. (2007, June 18). Countdown to coverage. *Boston Globe*, p. C-1.

Ehrenreich, B., & Ehrenreich, J. (1971). *The American health empire: Power, profits, and politics.* New York: Random House, Vintage Books. (The headings that follow this reference in the text are quoted from this book.)

Harris, G., Carey, B., & Roberts, J. (2007, May 10). Psychiatrists, troubled children, and drug industry's role. *New York Times*, p. A1.

Kassirer, J. P. (2005). *On the take.* New York: Oxford University Press.

Knowles, J. (1970, January). It's time to operate. *Fortune*, p. 79.

Kowalczyk, L. (2007a, March 25). At the ER, the stay can reach 8 hours. *Boston Globe*, p. A-1.

Kowalczyk, L. (2007b, April 21). Five hospitals release data on inspections. *Boston Globe*, p. A-1.

Kowalczyk, L. (2007c, September 17). Many Mass. hospitals will pay for errors. *Boston Globe*, p. A-1.

Meier, B. (2007, May 11). Narcotic maker guilty of deceit over marketing. *New York Times*, p. A1.

National Center for Health Statistics [NCHS]. (2006). *Health, United States, 2006 with chartbook on trends in the health of Americans.* Hyattsville, MD: Author.

National Center for Health Statistics. (2007). *Health, United States, 2007 with chartbook on trends in the health of Americans.* Hyattsville, MD: Author.

Saltus, R. (1999, February 18). Managed, yes, but couple wonders, is care? *Boston Globe*, p. A-1.

Saul, S. (2007, July 22). Drug safety crusader gets results, criticism. *Boston Globe*, p. A-6.

Smith, S. (2007, July 20). Tests of ER trainees find signs of race bias in care. *Boston Globe*, p. A-1.

Suchman, E. A. (1964). Sociomedical variations among ethnic groups. *American Journal of Sociology, 70,* 319–331.

Suchman, E. A. (1965). Social patterns of illness and medical care. *Journal of Health and Human Behavior, 6,* 2–16.

Torrens, P. R. (1988). Historical evolution and overview of health services in the United States. In S. J. Williams & P. R. Torrens (Eds.), *Introduction to health services* (3rd ed.). New York: John Wiley & Sons.

USA Today/Kaiser Family/Harvard School of Public Health. (2005, August). Menlo Park, CA: Henry J. Kaiser Family Foundation.

Zitner, A. (1999, March 14). Demographers caught looking on US trends. *Boston Sunday Globe*, A1.

Zola, I. K. (1996 October). Culture and symptoms: An analysis of patients presenting complaints. *American Sociological Review, 31,* 615–630.

Zola, I. K. (1972, November). Medicine as an institution of social control. *Sociological Review, 20*(4), 487–504. (The headings that follow this reference in the text are quoted from this article.)

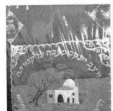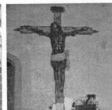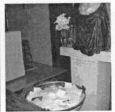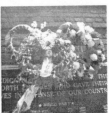

Chapter 5

HEALING Traditions

■ Objectives

1. Distinguish ways that one's religion influences HEALING.
2. Discuss the relationship of HEALING to today's health beliefs and practices.
3. Describe various forms of HEALING.
4. Differentiate rituals of birth and death among people of different religions.

The images in the chapter opener are representative of sacred places, shrines, from selected destinations of pilgrimages or spiritual tourism. These are places where people may travel to seek HEALTH or HEALING from deep within their traditional spiritual heritage or from a secular source of memory, solace, or HEALING. The first image is from the Tomb of Rachel in Bethlehem, Israel, and is a place where Jewish pilgrims may go seeking HEALTH protection, HEALING, and help, especially for fertility. People visit the Black Jesus in the San Fernando Cathedral in San Antonio, Texas, to petition for favors and HEALING and attest to countless miraculous HEALINGS. Petitions are placed at the Saint Ann's Shrine in Cleveland, Ohio. The last image represents the small secular shrines that may be set up at the scene of a fatal accident or at a memorial in a public setting, such as this one that is a veterans' memorial.

▨ HEALING

The professional history of nursing was born with Florence Nightingale's knowledge (1860) that "nature heals." In more recent times, Blattner (1981) has written a text designed to help nurses assist patients in upgrading their lives in a holistic sense and in healing the person—body, mind, and spirit. Krieger (1979), in *The Therapeutic Touch*, has developed a method for teaching nurses how to use their hands to heal. Wallace (1979) has described methods of helping nurses diagnose and deliver spiritual care. She points out that the word *spiritual* is often used synonymously with *religion* but that the terms are not the same. If they are used synonymously as a basis for the health care and nursing assessment of needs, some of the patient's deepest needs may be glossed over. *Spiritual care* implies a much broader grasp of the search for meanings that goes on within every human life. In addition to answers to these questions from nursing raised in the introduction to this chapter, one is able to explore the concept from the classical and historical viewpoints of anthropology, sociology, psychology, and religion.

From the fields of anthropology and sociology come texts that describe rituals, customs, beliefs, and practices that surround healing. Shaw (1975, p. 121) contends that, "for as long as man has practiced the art of magic, he has sought to find personal immortality through healing practices." Buxton (1973) describes traditional beliefs and indigenous HEALING rituals in Mandari and relates the source of these rituals with how humans view themselves in relation to God and Earth. In this culture, the healer experiences a religious calling to become a healer. HEALING is linked to beliefs in evil and the removal of evil from the sick person. Naegele (1970, p. 18) describes healing in our society as a form of "professional practice." He asserts, however, that "healing is not wholly a professional monopoly and that there are several forms of nonprofessional healing such as the 'specialized alternatives.'" These include Christian Science and the marginally professional activities of varying legitimacy, such as chiropractic, folk medicine, and quackery. He states: "To understand modern society is to understand the tension between traditional patterns and self-conscious rational calculations devoted to the mastery of everyday life."

Literature from the field of psychology abounds with references to HEALING. Shames and Sterin (1978) describe the use of self-hypnosis to HEAL, and Progoff (1959), a depth psychologist, describes depth as the "dimension of wholeness in man." He has written extensively on how one's discovery of the inner self can be used for both HEALING and CREATION.

Krippner and Villaldo (1976, p. viii) contend that there is a "basic conflict between healing and technology" and that "the reality of miracles, of healing, of any significant entity that could be called God is not thought to be compatible with the reality of science." They further contend that healings are psychosomatic in origin and useful only in the sense of the placebo effect.

The literature linking religion to HEALING is bountiful. The primary source is the Bible (both the Old and New Testament) and prayers. Bishop (1967, p. 45) discusses miracles and their relationship to healing. He states that the "miracles must be considered in relation to the time and place in which they occur." He further describes faith and its relationship to healing and states that "something goes on in the process of faith healing." He also points out that healing "is the exception rather than the rule." HEALING through faith generally is not accepted as a matter of plain fact, but it is an event to rejoice over.

Ford (1971, p. 6) describes healing of the spirit and methods of spiritual healing for spiritual illness. He describes suffering in three dimensions: body, mind, and spirit. He fully describes telotherapy—spiritual healing—which is both a means and an invitation. His argument is that full healing takes place only when there is agape love—divine love—and no estrangement from God. Russell (1937, p. 221) and Cramer (1923, p. 11) assert that healing is the work of God alone. Russell asserts that "God's will normally expresses itself in health," and Cramer focuses on the unity of human beings with God and claims that permanent health is truth, that healing is the gift of Jesus, and that it is a spiritual gift.

▨ Religion and HEALING

Religion plays a vital role in one's perception of HEALTH and ILLNESS. Just as culture and ethnicity are strong determinants in an individual's interpretation of the environment and the events within the environment, so, too, is religion. In fact, it is often difficult to distinguish between those aspects of a person's belief system arising from a religious background and those that stem from an ethnic and cultural heritage. Some people may share an ethnicity yet be of different religions; a group of people can share a religion yet have a variety of ethnic and cultural backgrounds. It is never safe to assume that all individuals of a given ethnic group practice or believe in the same religion. The point was embarrassingly driven home when I once asked a Chicano woman if she would like me to call the priest for her while her young son was awaiting a critical operation. The woman became angry with me. I could not understand why until I learned that she was a Methodist and not a Catholic. I had made an assumption, and I was wrong. She later told me that not all Chicanos are Catholic. After many years of hearing people make this assumption, she had learned to react with anger.

Religion strongly affects the way people interpret and respond to the signs and symptoms of ILLNESS. So pervasive is religion that the diets of many people are determined by their religious beliefs. Religion and the piety of a person determine not only the role that faith plays in the process of recovery but also in many instances the response to a given treatment and to the HEALING process. Each of these threads—religion, ethnicity, and culture—is woven into the fabric of each person's response to treatment and HEALING.

There are far too many religious beliefs and practices related to HEALING to include in this chapter. An introductory discussion of religious HEALING beliefs from the Judeo-Christian background, however, is possible.

The Old Testament does not focus on HEALING to the extent the New Testament does. God is seen to have total power over life and death and is the HEALER of all human woes. God is the giver of all good things and of all misfortune, including sickness. Sickness represented a break between God and humans. In Exodus 15:26, God is proclaimed the supreme HEALER ("I will put none of the diseases upon you which I put upon the Egyptians; for I am the Lord, your healer.") In a passage from Deuteronomy 32:39, it is stated "I kill, and I make alive. I have wounded and I heal." The traditionalist Jew believes that the "HEALING of illness comes from God through the mediation of His 'messenger,' the doctor." The Jew who is ill combines hope for a cure with faith in God and faith in the doctor (Ausubel, 1964, pp. 192–195). A prayer is recited for HEALING each Sabbath and other times throughout the week, and people are invited to submit or speak the names of people for whom they are petitioning for a restoration of their HEALTH.

The HEALING practices of the Roman Catholic tradition include a variety of beliefs and numerous practices of both a preventive and a HEALING nature. For example, St. Blaise, an Armenian bishop who died in A.D. 316 as a martyr, is revered as the preventer of sore throats. The blessing of the throats on his feast day (February 3) derives from the tradition that he miraculously saved the life of a boy by removing a fishbone he had swallowed (*Monthly Missalette*, 1980, p. 38).

Table 5-1   Selected Religions' Responses to Health Events

Baha'i
"All healing comes from God."

Abortion	Forbidden
Artificial insemination	No specific rule
Autopsy	Acceptable with medical or legal need
Birth control	Can choose family planning method
Blood and blood products	No restrictions for use
Diet	Alcohol and drugs forbidden
Euthanasia	No destruction of life
Healing beliefs	Harmony between religion and science
Healing practices	Pray
Medications	Narcotics with prescription
	No restriction for vaccines
Organ donations	Permitted
Right-to-die issues	Life is unique and precious—do not destroy
Surgical procedures	No restrictions
Visitors	Community members assist and support

Buddhist Churches of America
"To keep the body in good health is a duty—
otherwise we shall not be able to keep our mind strong and clear."

Abortion	Patient's condition determines
Artificial insemination	Acceptable
Autopsy	Matter of individual practice
Birth control	Acceptable

(continued)

Table 5-1 *Continued*

Blood and blood products	No restrictions
	Family, community
Diet	Restricted food combinations
	Extremes must be avoided
Euthanasia	May permit
Healing beliefs	Do not believe in healing through faith
Healing practices	No restrictions
Medications	No restrictions
Organ donations	Considered act of mercy; if hope for recovery, all means may be taken
Right-to-die issues	With hope, all means encouraged
Surgical procedures	Permitted, with extremes avoided
Visitors	Family, community

Roman Catholicism
"The prayer of faith shall heal the sick, and the Lord shall raise him up."

Abortion	Prohibited
Artificial insemination	Illicit, even between husband and wife
Autopsy	Permissible
Birth control	Natural means only
Blood and blood products	Permissible
Diet	Use foods in moderation
Euthanasia	Direct life-ending procedures forbidden
Healing beliefs	Many within religious belief system
Healing practices	Sacrament of sick, candles, laying on of hands
Medications	May be taken if benefits outweigh risks
Organ donations	Justifiable
Right-to-die issues	Obligated to take ordinary, not extraordinary, means to prolong life
Surgical procedures	Most are permissible except abortion and sterilization
Visitors	Family, friends, priest
	Many outreach programs through church to reach sick

Christian Science

Abortion	Incompatible with faith
Artificial insemination	Unusual
Autopsy	Not usual; individual or family decide
Birth control	Individual judgment
Blood and blood products	Ordinarily not used by members
Diet	No solid food restrictions
	Abstain from alcohol and tobacco, some from tea and coffee (caffeine)
Euthanasia	Contrary to teachings
Healing beliefs	Accepts physical and moral healing
Healing practices	Full-time healing ministers
	Spiritual healing practiced

Table 5-1 *Continued*

Medications	None
	Immunizations/vaccines to comply with law
Organ donations	Individual decides
Right-to-die issues	Unlikely to seek medical help to prolong life
Surgical procedures	No medical ones practiced
Visitors	Family, friends, and members of the Christian Science community and Healers, Christian Science nurses

Church of Jesus Christ of Latter-day Saints

Abortion	Forbidden
Artificial insemination	Acceptable between husband and wife
Autopsy	Permitted with consent of next of kin
Birth control	Contrary to Mormon belief
Blood and blood products	No restrictions
Diet	Alcohol, tea (except herbal teas), coffee, and tobacco are forbidden
	Fasting (24 hours without food and drink) is required once a month
Euthanasia	Humans must not interfere in God's plan
Healing beliefs	Power of God can bring healing
Healing practices	Anointing with oil, sealing, prayer, laying on of hands
Medications	No restrictions; may use herbal folk remedies
Organ donations	Permitted
Right-to-die issues	If death inevitable, promote a peaceful and dignified death
Surgical procedures	Matter of individual choice
Visitors	Church members (Elder and Sister), family, and friends
	The Relief Society helps members

Hinduism
"Enricher, Healer of disease, be a good friend to us."

Abortion	No policy exists
Artificial insemination	No restrictions exist but not often practiced
Autopsy	Acceptable
Birth control	All types acceptable
Blood and blood products	Acceptable
Diet	Eating of meat is forbidden
Euthanasia	Not practiced
Healing beliefs	Some believe in faith healing
Healing practices	Traditional faith healing system
Medications	Acceptable
Organ donations	Acceptable
Right-to-die issues	No restrictions
	Death seen as "one more step to nirvana"

(continued)

Table 5-1 *Continued*

Surgical procedures	With an amputation, the loss of limb is seen as due to "sins in a previous life"
Visitors	Members of family, community, and priest support

Islam
"The Lord of the world created me—and when I am sick, He healeth me."

Abortion	Not accepted
Artificial insemination	Permitted between husband and wife
Autopsy	Permitted for medical and legal purposes
Birth control	Acceptable
Blood and blood products	No restrictions
Diet	Pork and alcohol prohibited
Euthanasia	Not acceptable
Healing beliefs	Faith healing generally not acceptable
Healing practices	Some use of herbal remedies and faith healing
Medications	No restrictions
Organ donations	Controversial; must be discussed with family
Right-to-die issues	Attempts to shorten life prohibited
Surgical procedures	Most permitted
Visitors	Family and friends provide support

Jehovah's Witnesses

Abortion	Forbidden
Artificial insemination	Forbidden
Autopsy	Acceptable if required by law
Birth control	Sterilization forbidden
	Other methods individual choice
Blood and blood products	Forbidden
Diet	Abstain from tobacco, moderate use of alcohol
Euthanasia	Forbidden
Healing beliefs	Faith healing forbidden
Healing practices	Reading Scriptures can comfort the individual and lead to mental and spiritual healing
Medications	Accepted except if derived from blood products
Organ donations	Forbidden
Right-to-die issues	Use of extraordinary means an individual's choice
Surgical procedures	Not opposed, but administration of blood during surgery is strictly prohibited
Visitors	Members of congregation and elders pray for the sick person

Judaism
"O Lord, my God, I cried to Thee for help and Thou has healed me."

Abortion	Therapeutic permitted; some groups accept abortion on demand; seek rabbinical consultation
Artificial insemination	Permitted

Table 5-1 *Continued*

Autopsy	Permitted under certain circumstances
	All body parts must be buried together—seek rabbinical consultation
Birth control	Permissible, except with orthodox Jews—seek rabbinical consultation
Blood and blood products	Acceptable
Diet	Strict dietary laws followed by many Jews—milk and meat not mixed; predatory fowl, shellfish, and pork products forbidden; kosher products only may be requested
Euthanasia	Active Euthanasia Prohibited—passive euthanasia—not prolonging life may be acceptable—nutrition a basic need—not withheld—seek rabbinic consultation
Healing beliefs	Medical care expected
Healing practices	Prayers for the sick
Medications	No restrictions
Organ donations	Complex issue; some practiced—seek rabbinic consultation
Right-to-die issues	Right to die with dignity
	If death is inevitable, no new procedures need to be undertaken, but those ongoing must continue
Surgical procedures	Most allowed
Visitors	Family, friends, rabbi, many community services

Mennonite

Abortion	Therapeutic acceptable
Artificial insemination	Individual conscience; husband to wife
Autopsy	Acceptable
Birth control	Acceptable
Blood and blood products	Acceptable
Diet	No specific restrictions
Euthanasia	Not condoned
Healing beliefs	Part of God's work
Healing practices	Prayer and anointing with oil
Medications	No restrictions
Organ donations	Acceptable
Right-to-die issues	Do not believe life must be continued at all cost
Surgical procedures	No restrictions
Visitors	Family, community

Seventh-day Adventists

Abortion	Therapeutic acceptable
Artificial insemination	Acceptable between husband and wife
Autopsy	Acceptable
Birth control	Individual choice
Blood and blood products	No restrictions

(continued)

Table 5-1 *Continued*

Diet	Encourage vegetarian diet
Euthanasia	Not practiced
Healing beliefs	Divine healing
Healing practices	Anointing with oil and prayer
Medications	No restrictions
	Vaccines acceptable
Organ donations	Acceptable
Right-to-die issues	Follow the ethic of prolonging life
Surgical procedures	No restrictions
	Oppose use of hypnotism
Visitors	Pastor and elders pray and anoint sick person
	Worldwide health system includes hospitals and clinics

Unitarian/Universalist Church

Abortion	Acceptable, therapeutic and on demand
Artificial insemination	Acceptable
Autopsy	Recommended
Birth control	All types acceptable
Blood and blood products	No restrictions
Diet	No restrictions
Euthanasia	Favor nonaction
	May withdraw therapies if death imminent
Healing beliefs	Faith healing: seen as "superstitious"
Healing practices	Use of science to facilitate healing
Medications	No restrictions
Organ donations	Acceptable
Right-to-die issues	Favor the right to die with dignity
Surgical procedures	No restrictions
Visitors	Family, friends, church members

Source: Adapted with permission from Andrews, M. M., & Hanson, P. A. (1995). Religion, culture, and nursing, In J. S. Boyle & M. M. Andrews (Eds.), *Transcultural concepts in nursing care* (2nd ed.) (pp. 371–406). Philadelphia: J. B. Lippincott. Used with permission.

HEALING and Today's Beliefs

It is not an accident or a coincidence that today, more so than in recent years, we are not only curious but vitally concerned about the ways of HEALING that our ancestors employed. Some critics of today's health care system choose to condemn it, with more vociferous critics, such as Illich (1975), citing its failure to create a utopia for humankind. It is obvious to those who embrace a more moderate viewpoint that diseases continue to occur and that they outflank our ability to cure or prevent them. Once again, many people are seeking the services of people who are knowledgeable in the arts of HEALING and folk medicine. Many patients may elect, at some point in their lives, more specifically during an ILLNESS, to use modalities outside the medical establishment. It is important to understand the HEALERS.

Types of HEALING

A review of HEALING and spiritual literature reveals that there are four types of HEALING:

1. **Spiritual** *HEALING.*When a person is experiencing an illness of the spirit, spiritual HEALING applies. The cause of suffering is personal sin. The treatment method is repentance, which is followed by a natural healing process.

2. **Inner** *HEALING.*When a person is suffering from an emotional (mental) illness, inner HEALING is used. The root of the problem may lie in the person's conscious or unconscious mind. The treatment method is to heal the person's memory. The HEALING process is delicate and sensitive and takes considerable time and effort.

3. **Physical** *HEALING.*When a person is suffering from a disease or has been involved in an accident that resulted in some form of bodily damage, physical HEALING is appropriate. Laying on hands and speaking in tongues usually accompany physical HEALING. The person is prayed over by both the leader and members of a prayer group.

4. **Deliverance, or exorcism.**When the body and mind are victims of evil from the outside, exorcism is used. In order to effect treatment, the person must be delivered, or exorcised, from the evil. The ongoing popularity of films such as *The Exorcist* gives testimony to the return of these beliefs. Incidentally, the priest who has lectured in my classes stated that he does not, as yet, lend credence to exorcisms; however, he was guarded enough not to discount it, either.

The people who HEAL, both in the past and in the present, often have been those who received the gift of HEALING from a "divine" source. Many receive this gift in a vision and have been unable to explain to others how they know what to do. Other HEALERS learned their skills from their parents. Most of the HEALERS with acquired skills are women, who subsequently pass their knowledge on to their daughters. People who use herbs and other preparations to remove the evil from the sick person's body are known as herbalists. Other HEALERS include bone setters and midwives, and although early humankind did not separate ILLS of the body from those of the mind, some HEALERS were more adept at solving problems by using early forms of "psychotherapy."

▓ Ancient Rituals Related to the Life Cycle

Today, just as it did in antiquity, religion also plays a role in the rites surrounding both birth and death. Many of the rituals that we observe at the time of birth and death have their origins in the practices of ancient human beings. Close your eyes for a few moments and picture yourself living thousands and thousands of years ago. There is no electricity, no running water, no bathroom, no plumbing. The nights are dark and cold. The only signs of the passage of time are the changing seasons and the apparent movement of the various planets and stars through the heavens. You are prey to all the elements, as well as to animals and the unknown. How do you survive? What sort of rituals and practices assist you in maintaining your equilibrium within this often hostile environment? It is from this milieu that many of today's practices sprang.

Generally speaking, three critical moments occur in the life of almost every human being: birth, marriage, and death (Morgenstern, 1966, p. 3). One needs to examine the events and rites that were attendant on birth and death in the past and to demonstrate how many of them not only are relevant to our lives today but also are still practiced. Rites related to marriage are not included in this text but certainly are related, in the long term, to a person's HEALTH.

Birth Rituals

In the minds of early human beings, the number of evil spirits far exceeded the number of good spirits, and a great deal of energy and time was devoted to thwarting these spirits. They could be defeated by the use of gifts or rituals or, when the evil spirits had to be removed from a person's body, with redemptive sacrifices. Once these evil spirits were expelled, they were prevented from returning by various magical ceremonies and rites. When a ceremony and an incantation were found to be effective, they were passed on through the generations. It has been suggested and supported by scholars that, from this primitive beginning, organized religion came into being. Today, many of the early rites have survived in altered forms, and we continue to practice them.

The power of the evil spirits was believed to endure for a certain length of time. The 3rd, 7th, and 40th days were the crucial days in the early life of a child and the new mother. Hence, it was on these days, or on the 8th day, that most of the rituals were observed. It was believed that, during this period, the newborn and the mother were at the greatest risk from the power of supernatural beings and thus in a taboo state. "The concept underlying taboo is that all things created by or emanating from a supernatural being are his, or are at least in his power" (Morgenstern, 1966, p. 31). The person was freed from this taboo by certain rituals, depending on the practices of a given community. When the various rites were completed and the 40 days were over, both the mother and child were believed to be redeemed from evil. The ceremonies that freed the person had a double character: They were partly magic and partly religious.

I have deliberately chosen to present the early practices of Semitic peoples because their beliefs and practices evolved into the Judaic, Christian, and Islamic religions of today. Because the newborn baby and mother were considered vulnerable to the threats of evil spirits, many rituals were developed to protect them. For example, in some communities, the mother and child were separated from the rest of the community for a certain length of time, usually 40 days. Various people performed precautionary measures, such as rubbing the baby with different oils or garlic, swaddling the baby, and lighting candles. In other communities, the baby and mother were watched closely for a certain length of time, usually 7 days. (During this time span, they were believed to be intensely susceptible to the effects of evil—hence, close guarding was in order.) Orthodox Jews still refer to the seventh night of life as the "watch night" (Morgenstern, 1966, pp. 22–30).

The birth of a male child was considered more significant than that of a female, and many rites were practiced in observance of this event. One ritual sacrifice was cutting off a lock of the child's hair and then sprinkling his forehead with sheep's blood. This ritual was performed on the eighth day of life and may be practiced today among Muslims. In other Semitic countries, when a child was named, a sheep was sacrificed and asked to give protection to the infant. Depending on regional or tribal differences, the mother might be given parts of the sheep. It was believed that, if this sacrificial ritual was not performed on the 7th or 8th day of life, the child would die (Morgenstern, 1966, p. 87). The sheep's skin was saved, dried, and placed in the child's bed for 3 or 4 years as protection from evil spirits.

Both the practice of cutting a lock of a child's hair and the sacrifice of an animal served as a ceremony of redemption. The child could also be redeemed from the taboo state by giving silver—the weight of which equaled the weight of the hair—to the poor. Although not universally practiced, these rites are still observed in some form in some communities of the Arab world.

Circumcision is closely related to the ceremony of cutting the child's hair and offering it as a sacrifice. Some authorities hold that the practice originated as a rite of puberty: a body mutilation performed to attract the opposite sex. (Circumcision was practiced by many peoples throughout the ancient world. Alex Haley's *Roots* describes it as a part of initiating boys into manhood in Africa.) Other sources attribute circumcision to the concept of the sanctity of the male organ and claim that it was derived from the practice of ancestor worship. The Jews of ancient Israel, as today, practiced circumcision on the 8th day of life. The Muslims circumcise their sons on the 7th day in the tradition that Mohammed established. In other Muslim countries, the ritual is performed anywhere from the 10th day to the 7th year of life. Again, this sacrifice redeemed the child from being taboo in his early stages of life. Once the sacrifice was made, the child entered the period of worldly existence. The rite of circumcision was accompanied by festivals of varying durations. Some cultures and kinship groups feasted for as long as a week.

The ceremony of baptism is also rooted in the past. It, too, symbolically expels the evil spirits, removes the taboo, and is redemptive. It is practiced mainly among members of the Christian faith, but the Yezidis and other non-Christian sects also perform the rite. Water was thought to possess magical powers and was used to cleanse the body from both physical and spiritual maladies, which included evil possession and other impurities. Usually, the child was baptized on the 40th day of life. In some communities, however, the child was baptized on the 8th day. The 40th (or 8th) day was chosen because the ancients believed that, given performance of the particular ritual, this day marked the end of the evil spirits' influence (Morgenstern, 1966).

Some rituals also involved the new mother. For example, not only was she (along with her infant) removed from her household and community for 40 days, but in many communities she had to practice ritual bathing before she could return to her husband, family, and community. Again, these practices were not universal, and they varied in scope and intensity from people to people.

Extensions of Birth Rituals to Today's Practices

Early human beings, in their quest for survival, strove to appease and prevent the evil spirits from interfering with their lives. Their beliefs seem simple and naive, yet the rituals that began in those years have evolved into those that exist today. Attacks of the evil spirits were warded off with the use of amulets, charms, and the like. People recited prayers and incantations. Because survival was predicated on people's ability to appease evil spirits, the prescribed rituals were performed with great care and respect. Undoubtedly, this accounts in part for the longevity of many of these practices through the ages. For example, circumcision and baptism still exist, even when the belief that they are being performed to release the child from a state of being taboo may not continue to be held. It is interesting also that adherence to a certain timetable is maintained. For example, as stated, the Jewish religion mandates that the ritual of circumcision be performed on the 8th day of life as commanded by Jewish law in the Bible.

The practice of closely guarding the new mother and baby through the initial hours after birth is certainly not foreign to us. The mother is closely watched for hemorrhage and signs of infection; the infant initially is watched for signs of choking or respiratory distress. This form of observation is very intense. Could factors such as these have been what our ancestors watched for? If early human beings believed that evil spirits caused the frequent complications that surrounded the birth of a baby, it stands to reason that they would seek to control or prevent these complications by adhering to astute observation, isolation, and rituals of redemption.

Death Rituals

It was believed that the work of evil spirits and the duration of their evil— whether it was 7 or 40 days—surrounded the person, family, and community at the time of and after death. Rites evolved to protect both dying and dead persons and the remaining family from these evil spirits. The dying person was cared for in specific ways (ritual washing), and the grave was prepared in set ways (storing food and water for the journey·after death). Further rituals were performed to protect the deceased's survivors from the harm believed to be rendered by the deceased's ghost. It was believed that this ghost could return from the grave and, if not carefully appeased, harm surviving relatives (Morgenstern, 1966, pp. 117–160).

Countless ethnocultural and religious differences can be found in the ways we observe dying, death, and mourning. The expressions for death have been collected over several years of randomly reading the local newspapers' death notices. It is interesting to observe the regional differences in expressions and that in some locations deaths are merely listed by the person's name and in other locations the event of death evokes comments such as "sunrise. . . sunset" and "departed this life."

Expressions of death and death rituals are also found in objects.

- Masks represent methods people use to hide from the "Angel of Death." Masks may also be placed on the face of the deceased.
- A bride and groom skeleton convey the message that marriage is forever, even unto death. The souls of the bride and groom are united for eternity.
- Candles are used by many people after a death as a way of lighting the way for the soul of the deceased.
- Jade stone, from China, is placed in orifices of the body to block the entrance of evil spirits after death.
- Ghost money, from China, is burned to send payments to a deceased person and to ensure his or her well-being in the afterlife.

Intersections of HEALTH, HEALING, and RELIGION

There are several areas in which there is an intersection of HEALTH, HEALING, and RELIGION. One's religious affiliation may be seen as providing many links in a complex chain of life events. Religious affiliation frequently provides a background for a person regarding HEALTHY behavior and contributes to HEALTH. Participation in religious practices provides social support and this in turn brings HEALTH. In addition, religious worship may create positive emotions; this, too, contributes to HEALTH. Table 5–2 illustrates several of these intersections, which must be known by health care providers.

This chapter has been no more than an overview of the topics introduced. The amount of relevant knowledge could fill many books. The issues raised here are those that have special meaning to the practice of nursing, medicine, and health care delivery. We must be aware (1) of what people are thinking that may differ from our own thoughts and (2) that sources of help exist outside the modern medical community. As the beliefs of ethnic communities are explored in later chapters, the text discussions will attempt to delineate who are specifically recognized and used as HEALERS by the members of the communities, and will describe some of the forms of treatment used by each community.

Table 5-2 **Areas of Intersection Between the Provision of Health Care and HEALTH, HEALING, and RELIGION**

Communication	Spirituality and religion begin in silence; however, the need for adequate interpreters has been addressed, but it is also imperative to have available to people the members and leaders of their faith community who can reach out and interpret what is happening in regard to a health crisis at a deeper and spiritual level for the patient and family
Gender	Understand the "rules" for gender care; in many faith traditions—for example, among Orthodox Jews and Muslims—care must be gender-specific and people of opposite genders may be forbidden to be touched by someone of the opposite gender
Modesty	Religious and elderly people may be extremely modest and modesty *must* be safe-guarded at all times
Diet	There are many food taboos predicated by one's religion and consideration must be given to see that improper foods are not served to patients
Objects	Sacred objects, such as amulets and statues, must be allowed in the patient's space and all precautions must be observed to safeguard them
Social organization	Spirituality or a religious background contributes many positive factors to the health care situation; collaboration with the leaders of a faith community can result in strongly positive outcomes for a patient and family
Space	Space must be defined and allocated for the patient's and family's private use
Time	Health care providers must be knowledgeable about sacred time—for example, what day the patient and family observe as a day of rest—Friday for Muslims, Friday sunset until Saturday sunset for Jews and Seventh-day Adventists, and Sunday for Christians; calendars must be posted that note holidays for all the faith traditions of people served within a given institution; meetings should not be held on these dates; Appendix B contains a list of religious holidays that do not occur on the same date each year; clergy within the faith tradition must be contacted to provide the dates for the holidays on a yearly basis

Explore 🌐 MediaLink

Go to the Companion Website at www.prenhall.com/spector for chapter-related review questions, case studies, and activities. Contents of the CulturalCare Guide and CulturalCare Museum can also be found on the Companion Website. Click on Chapter 5 to select the activities for this chapter.

Internet Sources

Fatima, A grace for Mankind. (2006). http://www.ewtn.com/fatima

Lourdes-France.org. (2008). Numerous links to information and history of the site. Lourdes, France: Author. Retrieved March 2, 2008 from http://www.lourdesfrance.org/index.php?goto_centre=ru&contexte=en&id=405

The University of Texas at Brownsville and Texas Southmost University. (2006). *El Nino Fidencio, Curanderismo* Research Project. Brownsville, Texas: Author. Retrieved March 1, 2008 from http://vpea.utb.edu/elnino/fidencio.html

References

Ausubel, N. (1964). *The book of Jewish knowledge*. New York: Crown.

Bishop, G. (1967). *Faith healing: God or fraud?* Los Angeles: Sherbourne.

Blattner, B. (1981). *Holistic nursing*. Englewood Cliffs, NJ: Prentice Hall.

Buxton, J. (1973). *Religion and healing in Mandari*. Oxford: Clarendon.

Cramer, E. (1923). *Divine science and healing*. Denver: The Colorado College of Divine Science.

Ford, P. S. (1971). *The healing trinity: Prescriptions for body, mind, and spirit*. New York: Harper & Row.

Foy, F. A. (Ed.). (1980). *Catholic almanac*. Huntington, IN: Our Sunday Visitor.

Gardner, D. (1992). *Niño Fidencio: A heart thrown open*. Santa Fe: Museum of New Mexico Press.

Geissler, E. M. (1994). *Pocket guide: Cultural assessment*. St. Louis: Mosby.

Geissler, E. M. (1998). *Pocket guide: Cultural assessment* (2nd ed.). St. Louis: Mosby.

Hallam, E. (1994). *Saints*. New York: Simon & Schuster.

Illich, I. (1975). *Medical nemesis: The expropriation of health*. London: Marion Bogars.

Informational brochure. (1953). *Shrine of Our Lady of La Leche*. St. Augustine, FL, (personal visit, 1999).

Informational brochure. (1999). *Shrine of the Blessed Virgin Mary*. Christ of the Hills Monastery, Blanco, TX, (personal visit, 1997).

Informational brochure. (n.d.). *Chimayo, New Mexico, the Shrine of our Lord of Esquipulas*.

Johnson, C. J., & McGee, M. G. (Eds.). (1991). *How different religions view death and afterlife*. Philadelphia: Charles Press.

Kelsey, M. T. (1973). *Healing and Christianity*. New York: Harper & Row.

Krieger, D. (1979). *The therapeutic touch*. Englewood Cliffs, NJ: Prentice Hall.

Krippner, S., & Villaldo, A. (1976). *The realms of healing*. Millbrae, CA: Celestial Arts.

Lipson, J. G., Dibble, S. L., & Minarik, P. A. (1996). *Cultural and nursing care: A pocket guide*. San Francisco: UCSF Nursing Press.

Monthly Missalette, 15(13) (1980, February), 38.

Morgenstern, J. (1966). *Rites of birth, marriage, death and kindred occasions among the Semites*. Chicago: Quadrangle Books.

Naegele, K. (1970). *Health and healing*. San Francisco: Jossey-Bass.

Nightingale, F. (1860, 1946). (A facsimile of the first edition published by ·D. Appleton and Co.). *Notes on nursing—What it is, what it is not.* New York: Appleton-Century.

Progoff, I. (1959). *Depth psychology and modern man.* New York: McGraw-Hill.

Russell, A. J. (1937). *Healing in his wings.* London: Methuen.

Shames, R., & Sterin, C. (1978). *Healing with mind power.* Emmaus, PA: Rodale Press.

Shaw, W. (1975). *Aspects of Malaysian magic.* Kuala Lumpur, Malaysia: Nazibum Negara.

Wallace, G. (1979, November). Spiritual care—A reality in nursing education and practice. *The Nurses Lamp, 5*(2), 1–4.

Unit

III

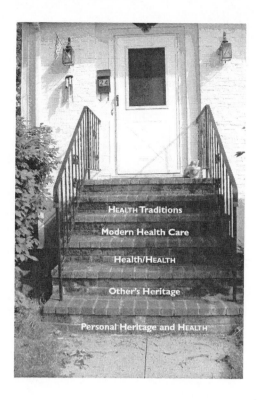

HEALTH Traditions

Modern Health Care

Health/HEALTH

Other's Heritage

Personal Heritage and HEALTH

HEALTH and ILLNESS Panoramas

The five chapters in this unit embrace the fifth step—traditional HEALTH care—and will provide a framework for learning about the communities you may be practicing in. It presents examples of the *traditional* HEALTH, ILLNESS, and HEALING beliefs and practices of selected populations. Each chapter introduces the

- Background of the population
- *Traditional* definitions of HEALTH/ILLNESS/HEALING
- *Traditional* methods of HEALTH maintenance and protection
- *Traditional* methods of HEALTH restoration
- Current health problems
- Health disparities in morbidity and mortality rates and in manpower

These are areas that can be applied in researching information regarding the populations you are caring for and working with. The World Wide Web is extremely helpful in gathering the demographic and modern health-related data applicable to a given population.

The need for historical, pertinent, and compelling information was recently driven home when I was discussing New Year's Day with a cohort of fifteen 21-year-old college senior students. The students did not know that New Year's Day—January 1—is a religious holiday; they believed it was a secular holiday. The conversation that resulted from this incident revealed a "thirst" for knowledge regarding *tradition*. They were eager to learn about the HEALTH traditions and other cultural events from their own ethnocultural heritage, from the heritages of peers, and the heritages of other people. Thus, an effort has been exerted to maintain the integrity of older references and the primary data that have been gathered regarding HEALTH beliefs and practices over the 30 years I have developed this text. In the race to modernity, science, technology, and "scholarly" endeavors, the HEALTH traditions of family and others may well be lost—as the saying goes, the baby was "thrown away with the bath water," to this generation.

The chapters in Unit III will present an overview of relevant historical and contemporary theoretical content that will help you

1. Develop a level of awareness of the background and health/HEALTH problems of both the emerging majority and White ethnic populations.
2. Understand and describe selected *traditional* HEALTH beliefs and practices.
3. Understand the *traditional* pathways to HEALTH care and the relationship between these pathways and the American health care system.
4. Understand certain manpower problems of each of the communities discussed.
5. Be more familiar with the available literature regarding each of the communities.

The following exercises are appropriate to all chapters in Unit III:

1. Familiarize yourself with some literature of the given community—that is, read literature, poetry, or a biography of a member of each of the communities.
2. Familiarize yourself with the history and sociopolitical background of each of the communities.

The questions that follow should be thoughtfully considered:

1. What are the traditional definitions of *HEALTH* and *ILLNESS* in each of the communities? Are they alike or different?
2. What are the traditional methods of maintaining HEALTH?
3. What are the traditional ways of protecting HEALTH?
4. What are the traditional ways of restoring HEALTH?
5. Who are the traditional HEALERS? What functions do they perform?

This is an extraordinary way to build connections between communities and to see how much different ethnocultural and religious communities have in common. Since HEALTH is the metaphor for this text, it brings to the forefront a way to analyze and understand some of the variability in health care.

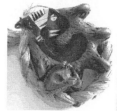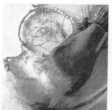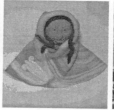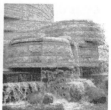

Chapter 6

HEALTH and ILLNESS in the American Indian and Alaska Native Population

Everything on the earth has a purpose, every disease an herb to cure it, and every person a mission. This is the Indian theory of existence.

—*Morning Dove (Christine Quintasket) (1888–1936) Salish*

■ Objectives

1. Discuss the background of the American Indian and Alaska Native population.
2. Describe the traditional definitions of HEALTH and ILLNESS of the American Indian and Alaska Native population.
3. Describe the traditional methods of HEALING of the American Indian and Alaska native population.
4. Describe the practice of a traditional healer.
5. Describe current health care problems of the American Indian and Alaska Native population.

The images opening this chapter portray items that may be used or places visited by people of a North American Indian heritage. The bear and bear claw represent sacred symbols of an animal that is revered and sacred to many people. The bear is symbolic of the power of nature. The drawstring bag is symbolic of the tobacco bag one may carry; tobacco is a sacred plant. The sweet grass surrounding the claw is from the American Indian Sioux Nation. It is burned, the flame is blown out, and the smoke is used to purify a room or home. The dreamcatcher in the second image is from the Cherokee Nation in Carolina. Traditional lore says that, if you keep this dreamcatcher near you, it will filter out ILLNESS and keep you well. The medicine bag from the Acama Pueblo in New Mexico holds herbs used in restoring HEALTH. The figure in the third image is a Cherokee house minder. It is the spirit of the little people, who are mischievous and enjoy playing tricks on the people who live in the home. They protect the home while the residents are away. The last image is a corner of the National Museum of the American Indian, which is a part of the Smithsonian Institution in Washington, DC. The exhibits change frequently and present images of American Indian life and culture. If you have not visited this museum, or the ones in New York City or Maryland, visit the Web site for a preview of the outstanding exhibits.

To realize the plight of today's American Indian, it is necessary to journey back in time to the years when Whites settled in this land. Before the arrival of Europeans, this country had no name but was inhabited by groups of people who called themselves nations. The people were strong both in their knowledge of the land and in their might as warriors. The Vikings reached the shores of this country about A.D. 1010. They were unable to settle on the land and left after a decade of frustration. Much later, another group of settlers, since termed the "Lost Colonies," were repulsed. More people came to these shores, however, and the land was taken over by Europeans.

As the settlers expanded westward, they signed "treaties of peace" or "treaties of land cession" with the American Indians. These treaties were similar to those struck between nations, although in this case the agreement was imposed by the "big" nation onto the "small" nation. One reason for treaties was to legitimize the takeover of the land that the Europeans had "discovered." Once the land was "discovered," it was divided among the Europeans, who set out to create a "legal" claim to it. The American Indians signed the resultant treaties, ceding small amounts of their land to the settlers and keeping the rest for themselves. As time passed, the number of Whites rapidly grew, and the number of Indians diminished because of wars and disease. As these events occurred, the treaties began to lose their meaning; the Europeans disregarded them. They decided that these "natives" had no real claim to the land and shifted them around like cargo from one reservation to another. Although the American Indians tried to seek just settlements through the American court system, they failed to win back the land that had been taken from them through misrepresentation. For example, in 1831, the Cherokees were fighting in the courts to keep their nation in Georgia. They lost their legal battle, however, and, like other American Indian nations after the time of the early European settlers, were forced to move westward. During this forced westward movement, many died, and all suffered. Today, many nations are seeking to reclaim their land through the courts (Brown, 1970; Deloria 1969, 1974; Fortney, 1977). Several claims, such as those of the Penobscot and Passamaquody tribes in Maine, have been successful. The number of federally recognized tribes has increased from just over 100 as recently ago as the 1980s to 561 presently (IHS, 2007).

As the American Indians migrated westward, they carried with them the fragments of their culture. Their lives were disrupted, their land was lost, and many of their leaders and teachers perished, yet much of their history and culture somehow remained. Today, more and more American Indians are seeking to know their history. The story of the colonization and settlement of the United States is being retold with a different emphasis.

American Indians live predominantly in 26 states (including Alaska), with most residing in the western part of the country as a result of the forced westward migration. Although many American Indians remain on reservations and in rural areas, just as many people live in cities, especially on the West Coast. Oklahoma, Arizona, California, New Mexico, and Alaska have the largest numbers of American Indians (IHS, 2007). Today, more and more people are claiming to have American Indian roots.

▥ Traditional Definitions of HEALTH and ILLNESS

Although each American Indian nation or tribe had its own history and belief system regarding HEALTH and ILLNESS and the traditional treatment of ILLNESS, some general beliefs and practices underlie the more specific tribal ideas. The terms HEALTH and ILLNESS are used to indicate that, among traditional people, the connotations are holistic. The data—collected through an ongoing review of the literature and from interviews granted by members of the groups—come from the Navajo Nation, Hopis, Cherokees, Shoshones, and New England Indians with whom I have worked closely.

The traditional American Indian belief about HEALTH is that it reflects living in "total harmony with nature and having the ability to survive under exceedingly difficult circumstances" (Zuckoff, 1995). Humankind has an intimate relationship with nature (Boyd, 1974). The Earth is considered to be a living organism—the body of a higher individual, with a will and a desire to be well. The Earth is periodically HEALTHY and less HEALTHY, just as human beings are. According to the American Indian belief system, a person should treat his or her body with respect, just as the Earth should be treated with respect. When the Earth is harmed, humankind, is itself harmed and, conversely, when humans harm themselves, they harm the Earth. The Earth gives food, shelter, and medicine to humankind; for this reason, all things of the Earth belong to human beings and nature. "The land belongs to life, life belongs to the land, and the land belongs to itself." In order to maintain HEALTH, Indians must maintain their relationship with nature. "Mother Earth" is the friend of the American Indian, and the land belongs to the American Indian (Boyd, 1974).

According to American Indian belief, as explained by a medicine man, Rolling Thunder, the human body is divided into two halves, which are seen as plus and minus (yet another version of the concept that every whole is made of two opposite halves). There are also—in every whole—two energy poles: positive and negative. The energy of the body can be controlled by spiritual means.

It is further believed that every being has a purpose and an identity. Every being has the power to control him- or herself and, from this force and the belief in its potency, the spiritual power of a person is kindled (Boyd, 1974).

In all American Indian cultures, disease is associated with the religious aspect of society as supernatural powers are associated with the causing and curing of disease. Disease is conceived of in a wide variety of ways. It is believed to occur due to a lack of prevention, which is given by wearing or using charms; the presence of some material object that has intruded into the body via sorcery; or the absence of the free soul from the body (Lyon, 1996, pp. 60–61). One example of an amulet is *Duklij*, turquoise or green malachite that is believed to contain supernatural qualities that ward off the evil spirits and bring rain (Lyon, 1996, p. 68).

Many American Indians with traditional orientations believe there is a reason for every sickness or pain. They believe that ILLNESS is the price to be paid either for something that happened in the past or for something that will happen in the future. In spite of this conviction, a sick person must still be cared for. Everything is seen as being the result of something else, and this cause-and-effect relationship creates an eternal chain. American Indians do not generally subscribe to the germ theory of modern medicine. ILLNESS is something that must be. Even the person who is experiencing the ILLNESS may not realize the reason for its occurrence, but it may, in fact, be the best possible price to pay for the past or future event(s) (Boyd, 1974).

The Hopi Indians associate ILLNESS with evil spirits. The evil spirit responsible for an ILLNESS is identified by the medicine man, and the remedy for the malady resides in the treatment of the evil spirit (Leek, 1975, p. 16).

According to legend, the Navajo people originally emerged from the depths of the Earth—fully formed as human beings. Before the beginning of time, they existed with holy people, supernatural beings with supernatural powers, in a series of 12 underworlds. The creation of all elements took place in these underworlds, and there all things were made to interact in constant harmony. A number of ceremonies and rituals were created at this time for "maintaining, renewing, and mending this state of harmony" (Bilagody, 1969, p. 21).

When the Navajo people emerged from the underworlds, one female was missing. She was subsequently found by a search party in the same hole from which they had initially emerged. She told the people that she had chosen to remain there and wait for their return. She became known as death, sickness, and witchcraft. Because her hair was unraveled and her body was covered with dry red ochre, the Navajos today continue to unravel the hair of their dead and to cover their bodies with red ochre. Members of the Navajo Nation believe that "witchcraft exists and that certain humans, known as witches, are able to interact with the evil spirits. These people can bring sickness and other unhappiness to the people who annoy them" (Bilagody, 1969, p. 36).

Traditionally, the Navajos see ILLNESS, disharmony, and sadness as the result of one or more combinations of the following actions: "(1) displeasing the holy people; (2) annoying the elements; (3) disturbing animal and plant life; (4) neglecting the celestial bodies; (5) misuse of a sacred Indian ceremony; or

(6) tampering with witches and witchcraft" (Bilagody, 1969, p. 57). If disharmony exists, disease can occur. The Navajos distinguish between two types of disease: (1) contagious diseases, such as measles, smallpox, diphtheria, syphilis, and gonorrhea, and (2) more generalized ILLNESSES, such as "body fever" and "body ache." The notion that ILLNESS is caused by a microbe or another physiological agent is alien to the Navajos. The cause of disease, of injury to people or to their property, or of continued misfortune of any kind must be traced back to an action that should not have been performed. Examples of such infractions are breaking a taboo and contacting a ghost or witch. To the Navajos, the treatment of an ILLNESS, therefore, must be concerned with the external causative factor(s), not with the ILLNESS or injury itself (Kluckhohn & Leighton, 1962, pp. 192–193).

▪ Traditional Methods of HEALING

Traditional HEALERS

The traditional HEALER of Native America is the medicine man or woman, and American Indians, by and large, have maintained their faith in him or her over the ages. The medicine men and women are wise in the ways of the land and of nature. They know well the interrelationships of human beings, the Earth, and the universe. They know the ways of the plants and animals, the sun, the moon, and the stars. Medicine men and women take time to determine first the cause of an ILLNESS and then the proper treatment. To determine the cause and treatment of an ILLNESS, they perform special ceremonies, which may take up to several days.

A medicine man or woman is also known among many people as a *Kusiut*, a "learned one." The acquisition of full shamanic powers takes many years, often as many as 30 years of training before one has the ability to cure illness. The shaman's power is accumulated through solitary vision quests and fasts repeated over the years. The purification rituals include scrubbing oneself in freezing cold water and ingesting emetics (Lyon, 1996, p. 141).

As a specific example, Boyd describes the medicine man, Rolling Thunder—the spiritual leader, philosopher, and acknowledged spokesman of the Cherokee and Shoshone tribes—as being able to determine the cause of ILLNESS when the ILL person does not know it. The "diagnostic" phase of the treatment may take as long as 3 days. There are numerous causes of ILLNESS and a great number of reasons—good or bad—for having become ILL. These causes are of a spiritual nature. When modern physicians see a sick person, they recognize and diagnose only the physical illness. Medicine men and women, in contrast, look for the spiritual cause of the problem. To the American Indian, "every physical thing in nature has a spiritual nature because the whole is viewed as being essentially spiritual in nature." The agents of nature, herbs, are seen as spiritual helpers, and the characteristics of plants must be known and understood. Rolling Thunder states that "we are born with a purpose in life and we have to fulfill that purpose" (Boyd, 1974, pp. 124, 263). The purpose of the medicine man or woman is to cure, and their power is not dying out.

The medicine man or woman of the Hopis uses meditation in determining the cause of an ILLNESS and sometimes even uses a crystal ball as the focal point for meditation. At other times, the medicine man or woman chews on the root of jimsonweed, a powerful herb that produces a trance. The Hopis claim that this herb gives the medicine man or woman a vision of the evil that has caused a sickness. Once the meditation is concluded, the medicine man or woman is able to prescribe the proper herbal treatment. For example, fever is cured by a plant that smells like lightning; the Hopi phrase for fever is "lightning sickness" (Leek, 1975, p. 16).

The Navajo Indians consider disease to be the result of breaking a taboo or the attack of a witch. The exact cause is diagnosed by divination, as is the ritual of treatment. There are three types of divination: motion in the hand (the most common form and often practiced by women), stargazing, and listening. The function of the diagnostician is first to determine the cause of the ILLNESS and then to recommend the treatment—that is, the type of chant that will be effective and the medicine man or woman who can best do it. A medicine man or woman may be called on to treat obvious symptoms, whereas the diagnostician is called on to ascertain the cause of the ILLNESS. (A person is considered wise if the diagnostician is called first.) Often, the same medicine man or woman can practice both divination (diagnosis) and the singing (treatment). When any form of divination is used in making the diagnosis, the diagnostician meets with the family, discusses the patient's condition, and determines the fee.

The practice of motion in the hand includes the following rituals. Pollen or sand is sprinkled around the sick person, during which time the diagnostician sits with closed eyes and face turned from the patient. The HEALER's hand begins to move during a song. While the hand is moving, the diagnostician thinks of various diseases and various causes. When the arm begins to move in a certain way, the diagnostician knows that the right disease and its cause have been discovered. He or she is then able to prescribe the proper treatment (Wyman, 1966, pp. 8–14). The ceremony of motion in the hand also may incorporate the use of sand paintings. (These paintings are a well-known form of art.) Four basic colors are used—white, blue, yellow, and black—and each color has a symbolic meaning. Chanting is performed as the painting is produced, and the shape of the painting determines the cause and treatment of the ILLNESS. The chants may continue for an extended time (Kluckhohn & Leighton, 1962, p. 230), depending on the family's ability to pay and the capabilities of the singer. The process of motion in the hand can be neither inherited nor learned. It comes to a person suddenly, as a gift. It is said that people able to diagnose their own ILLNESSES are able to practice motion in the hand (Wyman, 1966, p. 14).

Unlike motion in the hand, stargazing can and must be learned. Sand paintings are often but not always made during stargazing. If they are not made, it is either because the sick person cannot afford to have one done or because there is not enough time to make one. The stargazer prays the star prayer to the star spirit, asking it to show the cause of the ILLNESS. During stargazing, singing begins and the star throws a ray of light that determines the cause of the patient's ILLNESS. If the ray of light is white or yellow, the patient will recover; if it is red, the ILLNESS is serious. If a white light falls on the patient's home, the person will recover; if the home is dark, the patient will die (Wyman, 1966, p. 15).

Listening, the third type of divination, is somewhat similar to stargazing, except that something is heard rather than seen. In this instance, the cause of the ILLNESS is determined by the sound that is heard. If someone is heard to be crying, the patient will die (Wyman, 1966, p. 16).

The traditional Navajos continue to use medicine men and women when an ILLNESS occurs. They use this service because, in many instances, the treatment they receive from the traditional HEALERS is better than the treatment they receive from the health care establishment. Treatments used by singers include massage and heat treatment, the sweatbath, and use of the yucca root—approaches similar to those common in physiotherapy (Kluckhohn & Leighton, 1962, p. 230).

The main effects of the singer are psychological. During the chant, the patient feels cared for in a deeply personal way as the center of the singer's attention, since the patient's problem is the reason for the singer's presence. When the singer tells the patient recovery will occur and the reason for the ILLNESS, the patient has faith in what is heard. The singer is regarded as a distinguished authority and as a person of eminence with the gift of learning from the holy people. He or she is considered to be more than a mere mortal. The ceremony—surrounded by such high levels of prestige, mysticism, and power—takes the sick person into its circle, ultimately becoming one with the holy people by participating in the sing that is held on the patient's behalf. The patient once again comes into harmony with the universe and subsequently becomes free of all ILLS and evil (Kluckhohn & Leighton, 1962, p. 232).

The religion of the Navajos is one of good hope when they are sick or suffer other misfortunes. Their system of beliefs and practices helps them through the crises of life and death. The stories that are told during ceremonies give the people a glimpse of a world that has gone by, which promotes a feeling of security because they see that they are links in the unbroken chain of countless generations (Kluckhohn & Leighton, 1962, p. 233).

Many Navajos believe in witchcraft, and, when it is considered to be the cause of an ILLNESS, special ceremonies are employed to rid the individual of the evil caused by witches. Numerous methods are used to manipulate the supernatural. Although many of these activities may meet with strong social disapproval, Navajos recognize the usefulness of blaming witches for ILLNESS and misfortune. Tales abound concerning witchcraft and how the witches work. Not all Navajos believe in witchcraft but, for those who do, it provides a mechanism for laying blame for the overwhelming hardships and anxieties of life.

Such events as going into a trance can be ascribed to the work of witches. The way to cure a "witched" person is through the use of complicated prayer ceremonies that are attended by, friends and relatives, who lend help and express sympathy. The victim of a witch is in no way responsible for being sick and is, therefore, free of any punitive action by the community if the ILLNESS causes the victim to behave in strange ways. However, if an incurably "witched" person is affected so that alterations in the person's established role severely disrupt the community, the victim may be abandoned (Kluckhohn & Leighton, 1962, p. 244). Box 6–1 presents selected beliefs of a traditional Cherokee medicine man.

 Box 6–1

Hawk Littlejohn, 1941–2000

I had the privilege of working with Hawk Littlejohn, a traditional medicine man, in 1979 at the Boston (Massachusetts) Indian Council. Thomas Crowe wrote in his obituary that Hawk Littlejohn "embraced tradition in the modern world. He was a native of Western North Carolina and a member of the Eastern Band of the Cherokee nation. He was unique both in his skills in the traditional methods of natural and psychological healing and in his sensitivity and concern for his fellow man." I interviewed him in June 1979. Here are several of his thoughts in his own words:

- A medicine man sees himself in my tribe as a person who is many, many things. Not just as a HEALER or not just as a priest. We like to see ourselves like the fingers on a hand. They are separated and work independently of the hand if requested to, but they're still part of the whole. And each one of these fingers can do different things. It's like when I go to visit a home and there is a child there who is suffering from malnutrition but in our medicine we're more interested in the cause not the symptom. So, I've left my role as a HEALER and a priest to a role that might turn out to be social or political to find out why the child is hungry, why this child is feeling this way. And that might be dealing with the tribal government or some kind of social situation. We elect to see ourselves as representatives of our people's needs.
- The medicine man or HEALER in my tribe is considered to be chosen by the Great Spirit. For a couple of years the medicine men check all children for unusual marks, it is not any particular mark on the body but something they consider very unusual as a sign. The unusual marks that were on me were Simian Creases, the line that goes across my hand. I'm told it is unusual to have one of these but to have two, one on each hand, is very unusual. I was perhaps two or three years old when I was chosen.
- As a child I was taught that there are three parts of us and the most obvious part is the physical aspect, then the second part is the intellectual part, and the third part is the spiritual aspect of a person. The physical is the tangible, the one we can see and touch and be with all the time. We go through acceptance of our physical being. This is what I have to walk the path of life with and I accept it for what it is. The intellectual aspect is the part that interprets things for you—dreams, visions, feelings, and what the spirit is saying to you. The spiritual aspect of a person of is the slowest and the last in

most cases to mature. The spiritual aspect is kept in harmony and in balance by the awareness that it is part of everything else. We believe that all life forms have a spirit and the relationship of man to all other beings that are alive is a spiritual one. When all three aspects are working together it is called balance and harmony, or the center of the earth.

- Let's say a student, for example, puts a lot of emphasis on the intellect and neglects the physical and the spiritual aspect of him, we believe that there are natural forces which always try to seek a balance. For instance, if you get a cut, you heal because it is natural to try to seek balance. We believe that there are many subtle things the Great Spirit made and very obvious things that the Great Spirit made like creatures like elephants, whales, and the obvious. And then much more subtle creatures like what you call germs and viruses and when we believe that when the Great Spirit created life, he created laws to govern life, that the wolf wouldn't eat the deer in one day, that there would be laws to govern these kinds of things. One of the laws was what we call a "skilly." It is a being or a creature and it has no good or bad. When a person neglects the spiritual and physical part for the intellect, and does not seek balance, the skilly comes in and one of the effects of the skilly is sickness and disease.
- One of the ways to treat people is indirectly. When I go to see people we talk about their corn and their lives and they talk about my corn and my life and then we get down to the reason why I am there. They don't tell me their physical symptoms. One of the things we've realized is that sickness isolates people from other people and the sickness has separated the person from the community and from his family. So we automatically try to make him or bring him back out of that isolation and one of the ways we do that is to include the family and friends in the HEALING process.
- In my tribe we have knowledge of about 500 different plants and use about 350 of them on a pretty regular basis. We see the plants as other life forms, but the commonality between all life forms is this spiritual aspect. We believe that each thing that is alive has a spirit and its spirit has a personality, so I use the spirit of the plant to cure another spirit—when the spirit of the sickness is not compatible with the spirit of the plant, the disease dissipates. We call the plants, plant people. My people's medicine started off as a trial and error, like most medicine did, using the plants. If you had a sickness that reminded them of a rabbit, for example, a plant that reminded them of a fox would be used to treat it.
- I think the solution to Indian problems is for Indian people to start identifying themselves. I see as a traditional person that one of the steps on this long journey is to gain pride and dignity in oneself. Naturally, I believe it is in traditionalism. Traditionalism is a philosophy, a way of life and living, a holistic sort of thing that we're a part of.

Traditional Remedies

American Indians practice an act of purification in order to maintain their harmony with nature and to cleanse the body and spirit. This is done by total immersion in water in addition to the use of sweatlodges, herbal medicines, and special rituals. Purification is seen as the first step in the control of consciousness, a ritual that awakens the body and the senses and prepares a person for meditation. The participants view it as a new beginning (Boyd, 1974, pp. 97–100).

The basis of therapy lies in nature, hence the use of herbal remedies. Specific rituals are to be followed when herbs are gathered. Each plant is picked to be dried for later use. No plant is picked unless it is the proper one, and only enough plants are picked to meet the needs of the gatherers. Timing is crucial, and the procedures are followed meticulously. So deep is their belief in the harmony of human beings and nature that the herb gatherers exercise great care not to disturb any of the other plants and animals in the environment (Boyd, 1974, pp. 101–136).

One plant of interest, the common dandelion, contains a milky juice in its stem and is said to increase the flow of milk from the breasts of nursing mothers. Another plant, the thistle, is said to contain a substance that relieves the prickling sensation in the throats of people who live in the desert. The medicine used to hasten the birth of a baby is called "weasel medicine" because the weasel is clever at digging through and out of difficult territory (Leek, 1975, p. 17).

The use of American Indian cures and herbal remedies continues to be popular. Among the Oneida Indians, the following remedies are used (Knox & Adams, 1988):

Illness	Remedy
Colds	Witch hazel, sweet flag
Sore throat	Comfrey
Diarrhea	Elderberry flowers
Headache	Tansy and sage
Ear infection	Skunk oil
Mouth sores	Dried raspberry leaves

Among the Micmac Indians of Canada, the following remedies have been reported to be used (Basque and Young, 1984):

Illness	Remedy
Warts	Juice from milkweed plant
Obesity	Spruce bark and water
Rheumatism	Juniper berries
Diabetes	Combination of blueberries and huckleberries
Insomnia	A head of lettuce a day
Diarrhea	Tea from wild strawberry

Drums are another source of treatment. HEALING ceremonies are accompanied by drumming, rattles, and singing. The noise consists of sounds that interfere with the negative work of the spirits of the disease. The rhythm of the drumming plays a role in altering human consciousness (Lyon, 1996, p. 67). "Drumming is essential in helping the shaman make the transition from an ordinary state of consciousness to the shamanistic state of consciousness" (p. 68). Quiet HEALING ceremonies are unheard of.

Current Health Care Problems

Today, American Indians are faced with a number of health-related problems and health disparities. Many of the old ways of diagnosing and treating illness have not survived the migrations and changing ways of life of the people. Because these skills often have been lost and because modern health care facilities are not always available, American Indian people are frequently caught in limbo when it comes to obtaining adequate health care. At least one third of American Indians exist in a state of abject poverty. With this destitution come poor living conditions and attendant problems, as well as diseases of the poor—including malnutrition, tuberculosis, and high maternal and infant death rates. Poverty and isolated living serve as further barriers that keep American Indians from using limited health care facilities even when they are available. Many of the illnesses that are familiar among White patients may manifest themselves differently in American Indian patients. As alluded to at the beginning of this chapter, suicide rates among the young are high—a rate that is more than three times that of the general population (Nieves, 2007, p. A-9). The traumas that the American Indians in the Plains States experienced over the past 175 years, such as the massacre at Wounded Knee, are part of the problem, as is the decimation of the land and culture.

Morbidity and Mortality

The American Indian and Alaska Native people have long experienced lower health status when compared with other Americans. Lower life expectancy and the disproportionate disease burden exist perhaps because of inadequate education, disproportionate poverty, discrimination in the delivery of health services, and cultural differences. These are broad quality-of-life issues rooted in economic adversity and poor social conditions.

American Indians and Alaska Natives born today have a life expectancy that is 2.4 years less than the U.S. population of all races (74.5 years to 76.9 years, respectively, American Indian and Alaska Native infants die at a rate of nearly 10 per every 1,000 live births, as compared to 7 per 1,000 for the U.S. population (2001–2003 rates). Given the higher health status enjoyed by most Americans, the lingering health disparities of American Indians and Alaska Natives are troubling. In trying to account for the disparities, health care experts, policymakers, and tribal leaders are looking at many factors that impact the health of Indian people, including the adequacy of funding for the American Indian health care delivery system (Indian Health Service [2007] Fact Sheet. Retrieved February 23, 2008, from http://www.INS.gov).

The American Indian and Alaska Native population has several characteristics different from the U.S. population that would impact assessing the cost for providing similar health services enjoyed by most Americans. The American Indian population is younger, because of higher mortality, than all other U.S. races. The IHS service population is predominately rural, which should suggest lower costs; however, the disproportionate incidence of disease and medical conditions experienced by the American Indian population raises the costs, which almost obliterates the lower cost offsets.

Mental Illness

The family in this population is often a nuclear family, with strong biological and large extended family networks. Children are taught to respect traditions, and community organizations are growing in strength and numbers. Many American Indians tend to use traditional medicines and HEALERS and are knowledgeable about these resources. People may frequently be treated by a traditional medicine man or woman. The sweatlodge and herbs are frequently used to treat mental symptoms. Several diagnostic techniques include the use of divination, conjuring, and stargazing.

"Ghost sickness" affects some American Indians. This mental health problem involves a preoccupation with death and the deceased and is associated with witchcraft. Symptoms include bad dreams, weakness, feelings of danger, loss of appetite, and confusion. *Pibloktoq* is a malady that afflicts some members of arctic and subarctic Eskimo communities. It is characterized by abrupt dissociative episodes, accompanied by extreme excitement, followed by convulsive seizures and coma (American Psychiatric Association, 1994).

Alcoholism is a major mental health problem among American Indians. A comparison of the 10 leading causes of death among American Indians/Alaska Natives and the general population reveals that unintentional injuries (#3), chronic liver disease and cirrhosis (#6), and suicide (#8) rank higher as causes of death than for the population at large. Each of these causes of death is related to mental health problems, including alcoholism.

Fetal Alcohol Syndrome

"My son will forever travel through a moonless night with only the roar of the wind for company" (Dorris, 1989, p. 264). This quote reflects on the tragedy of fetal alcohol syndrome, an affliction that affects countless American Indian children. A new study from the Substance Abuse and Mental Health Services Administration (SAMHSA) shows that American Indians and Alaska Natives continue to have higher rates of alcohol use and illicit drug use disorders than other racial groups.

The markings of fetal alcohol syndrome include

■ Abnormal growth in height, weight, and/or head circumference, including microcephaly

■ Central nervous system in behavioral and/or mental health problems, including learning disabilities and abnormal sleeping and eating patterns

■ Appearance with a specific pattern of recognizable deformities, such as the three key facial features a smooth philtrum, a thin vermillion border, and small palpebral fissures (Bertrand, Floyd, & Weber, 2005, p. 3)

An estimated 70,000 fetal alcohol children are born each year in the United States, many of whom are American Indians. The worldwide numbers vary, with a range of 0.2–1.5 cases per 1,000 live births being most frequently reported (Bertrand et al, 2005, p. 3). Dorris (1989, p. 231) further points out that the son of an alcoholic biological father is three times more likely to become an abusive drinker.

This problem has grown over time and the impact increases with each generation. Mortality and morbidity rates for American Indians are directly affected by alcohol abuse. Alcohol abuse is the most widespread and severe problem in the American Indian community. It is extremely costly to the people and underlies many of their physical, mental, social, and economic problems, and the problem is growing worse. Hawk Littlejohn, the medicine man of the Cherokee Nation, Eastern band, attributes this problem, from a traditional point of view, to the fact that American Indians have lost the opportunity to make choices. They can no longer choose how they live or how they practice their medicine and religion. He believes that, once people return to a sense of identification within themselves, they begin to rid themselves of this problem of alcoholism. Whatever the solution may be, the problem is indeed immense (Littlejohn, 1979 Interview).

Domestic Violence

Another problem related to alcohol abuse in the American Indian people is domestic violence, sexual abuse, and the battering of women. A battered woman is one who is physically assaulted by her husband, boyfriend, or another significant other. The assault may consist of a push; severe, even permanent injury; sexual abuse; child abuse; or neglect. Once the pattern of abuse is established, subsequent episodes tend to get worse. This abuse is not traditional in American Indian life but has evolved. True American Indian love is based on a tradition of mutual respect and the belief that men and women are part of an ordered universe the people should live in peace. In the traditional American Indian home, children were raised to respect their parents, and they were not corporally punished. Violence toward women was not practiced. In modern times, however, the sanctions and protections against domestic violence have decreased, and the women are far more vulnerable. Many women are reluctant to admit that they are victims of abuse because they believe that they will be blamed for the assault. Hence, the beatings continue. A number of services are available to women who are victims, such as safe houses and support groups. It is believed that the long-range solution to this problem lies in teaching children to love—to nurture children and give them self-esteem, to teach boys to love and respect women, and to give girls a sense of worth. Amnesty International calls sexual abuse against American Indian women a "Maze of Injustice." It is "the failure to protect Indigenous women from sexual violence in the USA." The disproportionate impact on American Indian women is derived from disparate communities that vary with respect to law enforcement, jurisdiction, and health care and support services (Grenier & Lockjer, 2007, p. 3).

Domestic violence has a profound effect on the community and on the family. A pattern of abuse is easily established. It begins with tension: The female attempts to keep peace but the male cannot contain himself, a fight erupts, and then the crisis arrives. The couple may make up, only to fight again. Attempts to help must be initiated, or the cycle escalates. The problem is extremely complex. Some of the services available to a household experiencing domestic violence include

1. Tribal health: direct services for physical and mental health
2. Law enforcement: police protection may be necessary
3. Legal assistance: assistance for immediate shelter and emergency food and transportation

Urban Problems

More than 50% of American Indians live in urban areas; for example, in Seattle, Washington, there are over 15,000 American Indians. Although this population is not particularly dense, its rates of diphtheria, tuberculosis, otitis media with subsequent hearing defects, alcohol abuse, inadequate immunization, iron-deficiency anemia, childhood developmental lags, mental health problems (including depression, anxiety, and coping difficulties), and caries and other dental problems are high. As in all dysfunctional families, problems arise that are related to marital difficulties and financial strain, which usually are brought about by unemployment and the lack of education or knowledge of special skills. The tension often is compounded further by alcoholism.

Between 5,000 and 6,000 American Indians live in Boston. They experience the same problems as American Indians in other cities, yet there is an additional problem. Few non-Indian residents are even aware that there is an American Indian community in that city or that it is in desperate need of adequate health and social services.

Health Care Provider Services

Some historical differences in health care relate to geographic locations. American Indians living in the eastern part of this country and in most urban areas are not covered by the services of the Indian Health Service, services that are available to American Indians living on reservations in the West. In 1923, tribal government—under the control of the Bureau of Indian Affairs—was begun by the Navajos, who established treaties with the U.S. government, but in the areas of health and education the United States did not honor these treaties. Health services on the reservations were inadequate. Consequently, the people were sent to outside institutions for the treatment of illnesses, such as tuberculosis and mental health problems. As recently as 1930, the vast Navajo lands had only seven hospitals with 25 beds each. Not until 1955 were American Indians finally offered concentrated services with modern physicians. Only since 1965 have more comprehensive services been available to the Navajos.

Cultural and Communication Problems

A factor that inhibits the American Indian use of White-dominated health services is a deep, cultural problem: American Indians suffer disease when they come into contact with White health care providers. American Indians feel uneasy because for too many years they have been the victim of haphazard care and disrespectful treatment. All too often, conflict arises between what the American Indians perceive their illness to be and what the physicians diagnose. American Indians, like most people, do not enjoy long waits in clinics; separation from their families; the unfamiliar, regimented environment of the hospital; or the unfamiliar behavior of the nurses and physicians, who often display demeaning and demanding attitudes. Their response to this treatment varies. Sometimes they remain silent; other times they leave and do not return. Many American Indians request that, if the ailment is not an emergency, they be allowed to see the medicine man or woman first and then receive treatment from a physician. Often, when a sick person is afraid of receiving the care of a physician, the medicine man or woman encourages the person to go to the hospital.

Health care providers must be aware of several factors when they communicate with American Indians. One is recognition of the importance of nonverbal communication. Often, American Indians observe providers and say very little. A patient may expect a provider to deduce the problem through instinct rather than by the extensive use of questions during history taking. In part, this derives from the belief that direct quoting is intrusive on individual privacy. When examining an American Indian with an obvious cough, a provider might be well advised to use a declarative statement—"You have a cough that keeps you awake at night"—and then allow time for the patient to respond to the statement.

It is American Indian practice to converse in a very low tone of voice. It is expected that the listener will pay attention and listen carefully in order to hear what is being said. It is considered impolite to say, "Huh?" or "I beg your pardon" or to give any indication that the communication was not heard. Therefore, an effort should be made to speak with patients in a quiet setting, where they will be heard more easily.

Note taking is taboo. Indian history has been passed through generations by means of verbal storytelling. American Indians are sensitive about note taking while they are speaking. When one is taking a history or interviewing, it may be preferable to use memory skills rather than to record notes. This more conversational approach may encourage greater openness between the patient and the provider.

Another factor to be considered is differing perceptions of time between the American Indian patient and the provider. Life on the reservation is not governed by the clock but by the dictates of need. When an American Indian moves from the reservation to an urban area, this cultural conflict concerning time often exhibits itself as lateness for appointments. One solution is the use of walk-in clinics.

Explore 🌐 MediaLink

Go to the Companion Website at www.prenhall.com/spector for chapter-related review questions, case studies, and activities. Contents of the CulturalCare Guide and CulturalCare Museum can also be found on the Companion Website. Click on Chapter 8 to select the activities for this chapter.

Internet Sources

Crowe, T. (2001). "Hawk Littlejohn embraced the traditional ways in the modern world." Smokey Mountain News. Retrieved from http://www.smokymountainnews.com/issues/1_01/1_17_01/front_littlejohn.shtml, July 21, 2007.

Grenier, D., and Lockjer, R. (2007). Domestic violence. http://www.ihs.gov/MedicalPrograms/MCH/M/obgyn0607_Feat.cfm#dv.

National Museum of the American Indian. (2008). Home Page. Washington, DC: Smithsonian http://www.nmai.si.edu/

Somnath, S., and Shipman, S. (2006). The rationale for diversity in the health professions: A review of the evidence. Washington, DC: U.S. Department of Health and Human Services Health Resources and Services Administration Bureau of Health Professions. http://www.hrsa.gov/

United States Department of Commerce, U.S. Census Bureau. Census 2000. (2002). Retrieved July 21, 2007 from http://www.census.gov/

United States Department of Health and Human Services, Health Resources and Services. (2004). The National Survey of Registered Nurses 2004 Documentation for the General Public Use File, 2006, Bureau of Health Professions Health Resources and Services Administration. HRSA/BHPr and the National Sample Survey of Registered Nurses. http://www.hrsa.gov/

United States Department of Health and Human Services, Indian Health Service, IHS. (2007). Fact Sheets Indian Population Trends, Indian Health Service Trends. Retrieved July, 2007 and February, 2008 from http://info.ihs.gov/

References

American Psychiatric Association. (1994). *Diagnostic and statistical manual of mental disorders* (4th ed.). Washington, DC: Author.

Basque, E. and Young, P. (1984). Personal Interviews, Boston Indian Council.

Bertrand, J., Floyd, R. L., Weber, M. K. (2005). Guidelines for identifying and referring persons with fetal alcohol syndrome. MMWR. V.54/RR-11.

Bilagody, H. (1969). An American Indian looks at health care. In R. Feldman & D. Buch (Eds.), *The Ninth Annual Training Institute for Psychiatrist-Teachers of Practicing Physicians*. Boulder, CO: WICHE, No. 3A30.

Boyd, D. (1974). *Rolling Thunder.* New York: Random House.

Brown, D. (1970). *Bury my heart at Wounded Knee.* New York: Holt.

Deloria, V., Jr. (1969). *Custer died for your sins.* New York: Avon Books.

Deloria, V., Jr. (1974). *Behind the trail of broken treaties.* New York: Delacorte.

Dorris, M. (1989). *The broken cord.* New York: Harper & Row.

Fortney, A. J. (1977, January 23). Has White man's lease expired? *Boston Sunday Globe,* pp. 8–30.

Kluckhohn, C., & Leighton, D. (1962). *The Navaho* (Rev. ed.). Garden City, NY: Doubleday.

Knox, M. E., & Adams, L. (1988). *Traditional health practices of the Oneida Indian.* Oshkosh: University of Wisconsin, College of Nursing.

Leek, S. (1975). *Herbs: Medicine and mysticism.* Chicago: Henry Regnery.

Littlejohn, Hawk. (1979). Personal Interview. Boston MA.

Lyon, W. S. (1996). *Encyclopedia of Native American healing.* New York: Norton.

National Center for Health Statistics. (2006). *Health, United States, 2006 with chartbook on trends in the health of Americans* (pp. 135, 140, 144, 149, 160, 244, 230, 227). Hyattsville, MD: Author.

National Center for Health Statistics. (2007). *Health, United States, 2007 with chartbook on trends in the health of Americans.* Hyattsville, MD: Author.

Nieves, E. (2007, June 9). Indian reservation reeling in weave of youth suicides and attempts. *New York Times,* p. A-9.

Ogunwole, S. H. (2002). *The American Indian and Alaska Native population: 2000. U.S. Census 2000.* Washington, DC: U.S. Department of Commerce.

Spector, R. (1992). Culture, ethnicity, and nursing. In P. Potter & A. Perry (Eds.), *Fundamentals of nursing* (3rd ed.). St. Louis: Mosby-Year Book.

Wyman, L. C. (1966). Navaho diagnosticians. In W. R. Scott & E. H. Volkhart (Eds.), *Medical care.* New York: John Wiley & Sons.

Zuckoff, M. (1995, April 18). More and more claiming American Indian heritage. *Boston Globe,* A8.

▓ Additional Readings

Bear, S., & Bear, W. (1996). *The medicine wheel.* New York: Fireside.

Catlin, G. (1993). *North American Indian portfolio.* Washington, DC: Library of Congress.

Neihardt, J. G. (1991—original 1951). *When the tree flowered.* Lincoln: University of Nebraska Press.

Neihardt, N. (1993). *The sacred hoop.* Tekamah, NE: Neihardt.

Neihardt, J. G. (1998—original 1961). *Black Elk speaks.* Lincoln: University of Nebraska Press.

Noble, M. (1997). *Sweet Grass: Lives of contemporary Native women of the Northeast.* Mashpee, MA: C. J. Mills.

Peltier, L. (1999). *Prison writings: My life is my sun dance.* New York: St Martin's Press.

Senier, S. (2001). *Voices of American Indian assimilation and resistance.* Norman: University of Oklahoma Press.

Wiebe, R., & Johnson, Y. (1998). *Stolen life—The journey of a Cree woman.* Athens: Ohio University Press.

Wolfson, E. (1993). *From the Earth to the sky.* Boston: Houghton Mifflin.

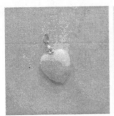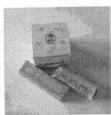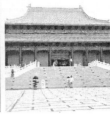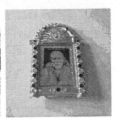

Chapter 7

HEALTH and ILLNESS in the Asian Populations

But when she arrived in the new country, the immigration officials pulled her swan away from her leaving the woman fluttering her arms and with only one swan feather for a memory.

—Amy Tan

■ Objectives

1. Discuss the background of the selected communities of the Asian populations.
2. Describe the traditional definitions of *HEALTH* and *ILLNESS* of selected communities of the Asian populations.
3. Describe the traditional methods of HEALING within selected communities of the Asian populations.
4. Describe current health care problems of members of selected communities of the Asian populations.

The images opening this chapter depict objects, substances, places, and people that people of Asian origins may use, visit, or beseech to protect, maintain, and/or restore HEALTH. Jade, from China, is believed to be the most precious of all stones. It is the giver of children, health, immortality, and wisdom. Jade charms are worn to bring HEALTH—to prevent harm and accidents—and in these ways to protect HEALTH. The two small boxes in the second section contain minute pills made of herbs used for stomach ailments and the larger box contains a large wax ball with a preparation of *Jen Shen Lu Jung Wan* (Ginseng antler pills) in it. These pills are used as a general tonic to strengthen the body and to improve digestion. The image in the third section is that of the *Hsi Lai* Buddhist Temple in Hacienda Heights, California. The massive temple was built in order to be a cultural and spiritual center and is the ideal of its founder, Venerable Master *Hsing Yun* to promote Humanistic Buddhism. The fourth section contains an icon with the image of the *Sai Baba*. He was a healer in India who continues to have a following of many people.

■ Background

The nearly 12 million people who constitute the Asian communities are the United States' third largest emerging majority group. This number included 10.2 million people, or 3.6% of total population, who reported only Asian and 1.7 million people, or 0.6%, who reported Asian as well as one or more other races. The term *Asian* refers to people having origins in any of the original peoples of the Far East, Southeast Asia, or the Indian subcontinent (for example, Cambodia, China, India, Japan, Korea, Malaysia, Pakistan, the Philippine Islands, Thailand, and Vietnam). The Asian groups are not limited to nationalities but are characterized by their diversity: More than 30 different languages are spoken and there is a similar number of cultures (Martin, 1995) and many different religions, including, but not limited to, Buddhism, Confucianism, Hinduism, Islam, and Taoism. The Asian population increased faster than the total population of the United States between 1990 and 2000. About one half (49%) of the Asian population lived in the West, 20% lived in the Northeast, 19% lived in the South, and 12% lived in the Midwest. Over half of all people who reported Asian lived in just three states: Hawaii, California, and Washington. The cities with the largest Asian populations are New York, Los Angeles, San Jose, San Francisco, and Honolulu (Barnes & Bennett, 2002, pp. 1–3, 7). There have been 8,226,255 people admitted from Asia since before 1980, 50.8% of whom have been naturalized; 1,192,435 people admitted from China, 50% of whom have been naturalized; and 1,022,550 people admitted from India, 38% of whom have been naturalized (U.S. Census Bureau, 2002).

Census 2000 designated the Native Hawaiian and other Pacific Islanders as a separate category. However, because the population is small, health data are not reported for this group alone. Therefore, the data related to the population are nested within this chapter. The population of Native Hawaiian and Other Pacific Islanders numbers 874,000, or 0.3%, of the total U.S. population. The term refers to people having origins in any of the original peoples of Hawaii, Guam,

Samoa, or other Pacific Islands. The people come from different cultures and speak many different languages (Grieco, 2001, pp. 1–2).

In Census 2000, the largest group of Asians was Chinese, with a total of 2.7 million people. Filipinos (2.4 million) and Asian Indians (1.9) were the next largest groups. Combined, Chinese, Filipinos, and Asian Indians account for 58% of the Asian population. Asian-born residents comprised 26% of the country's foreign-born population in 2000. Close to half of the nation's Asian-born population lived in one of three metropolitan areas—Los Angeles, New York, or San Francisco.

This chapter focuses on the traditional HEALTH and ILLNESS beliefs and practices of the Chinese and Indian Americans because those of many of the other Asians and Pacific Islanders are derived in part from the Chinese and Ayurvedic HEALTH traditions.

Chinese immigration to the United States began over 100 years ago. In 1850 there were only 1,000 Chinese inhabitants in this country; in 1880 there were well over 100,000. This rapid increase occurred in part because of the discovery of gold in California and in part because of the need for cheap labor to build the transcontinental railroads. The immigrants were laborers who met the needs of the dominant society. Like many early immigrant groups, they came here intending only to stay as temporary workers. Most of the immigrants were men, and they clung closely to their customs and beliefs and stayed together in their own communities. The hopes that many had for a better life when they came to the United States did not materialize. Subsequently, many of the workers and their kin returned to China before 1930. Part of the disharmony and disenchantment occurred because these immigrants were not White and did not have the same culture and habits as Whites. For these reasons, they were not welcomed, and many jobs were not open to them. For example, Chinese immigrant workers were excluded from many mining, construction, and other hard-labor jobs, even though the transcontinental railroad was constructed mainly by Chinese laborers. Between 1880 and 1930, the Chinese population declined by nearly 20%. One factor that helped perpetuate this decline in population was a series of exclusion acts halting further immigration. The people who remained behind were relegated to menial jobs, such as cooking and dishwashing. The Chinese workers first took these jobs in the West and later moved eastward throughout the United States. They tended to move to cities where they were allowed to let their entrepreneurial talents surface—their main pursuits included running small laundries, food shops, and restaurants.

The people settled in tightly knit groups in urban neighborhoods that took the name "Chinatown." Here they were able to maintain the ancient traditions of their homeland. They were hard workers and, in spite of the dull, menial jobs usually available to them, they were able to survive.

Both U.S. immigration laws and political problems in China have had an effect on the nature of today's Chinese population. When the exclusion acts were passed, many men were left alone in this country without the possibility that their families would join them. For this reason, a great majority of the men spent many years alone. In addition, the political oppression experienced by the Chinese in the United States was compounded—at a time when immigration laws were relaxed here after World War II, people were unable to return to or leave China because of that country's restrictive new regulations. By 1965, however, a large number of refugees who had relatives here were able to come to this country. They settled in the Chinatowns of America, causing the population of these areas to swell. The rate of increase since 1965 has been 10% per year.

▨ Traditional Definitions of *Health* and *Illness*

Chinese medicine teaches that HEALTH is a state of spiritual and physical harmony with nature. In ancient China, the task of the physician was to prevent ILLNESS. A first-class physician not only cured an ILLNESS but could also prevent disease from occurring. A second-class physician had to wait for patients to become ill before they could be treated. The physician was paid by the patient while the patient was healthy. When illness occurred, payments stopped. Indeed, not only was the physician not paid for services when the patient became ill, but the physician also had to provide and pay for the needed medicine (Mann, 1972, p. 222).

To understand the Chinese philosophy of HEALTH and ILLNESS, it is necessary to look back at the age-old philosophies from which more current ideas have evolved. The foundation rests in the religion and philosophy of Taoism. Taoism originated with a man named Lao-Tzu, who is believed to have been born about 604 B.C. The word *Tao* has several meanings: way, path, or discourse. On the spiritual level, it is the way of ultimate reality. It is the way of all nature, the primeval law that regulates all heavenly and earthly matters. To live according to the Tao, one must adapt oneself to the order of nature. Chinese medical works revere the ancient sages who knew the way and "led their lives in Tao" (Smith, 1958, pp. 175–192).

The Chinese view the universe as a vast, indivisible entity, and each being has a definite function within it. No one thing can exist without the existence of the others. Each is linked in a chain that consists of concepts related to each other in harmonious balance. Violating this harmony is like hurling chaos, wars, and catastrophes on humankind—the end result of which is ILLNESS. Individuals must adjust themselves wholly within the environment. Five elements—wood, fire, earth, metal, and water—constitute the guiding principles of humankind's surroundings. These elements can both create and destroy each other. For example, "wood creates fire," "two pieces of wood rubbed together produce a spark," "wood destroys earth," "the tree sucks strength from the earth." The guiding principles arise from this "correspondences" theory of the cosmos (Wallnöfer & von Rottauscher, 1972, pp. 12–16, 19–21).

For a person to remain HEALTHY, his or her actions must conform to the mobile cycle of the correspondences. The exact directions for achieving this were written in such works as the *Lu Chih Ch'un Ch'iu* (*Spring and Autumn Annals*) written by Lu Pu Wei, who died circa 230 B.C.

The holistic concept, as explained by Dr. P. K. Chan (1988), is an important idea of traditional Chinese medicine in preventing and treating diseases. It has two main components:

1. A human body is regarded as an integral organism, with special emphasis on the harmonic and integral interrelationship between the viscera and the superficial structures in these close physiological connections, as well as their mutual pathological connection. In Chinese medicine, the local pathological changes always are considered in conjunction with other tissues and organs of the entire body, instead of considered alone.

2. Special attention is paid to the integration of the human body with the external environment. The onset, evolution, and change of disease are considered in conjunction with the geographic, social, and other environmental factors.

Four thousand years before the English physician William Harvey described the circulatory system in 1628, *Huang-ti Nei Ching* (*Yellow Emperor's Book of Internal Medicine*) was written. This is the first known volume that describes the circulation of blood. It described the oxygen-carrying powers of blood and defined the two basic world principles: *yin* and *yang*, powers that regulate the universe. *Yang* represents the male, positive energy that produces light, warmth, and fullness. *Yin* represents the female, negative energy—the force of darkness, cold, and emptiness. *Yin* and *yang* exert power not only over the universe but also over human beings.

Yin and *yang* were further explained by Dr. Chan as having been originally a philosophical theory in ancient China. Later, the theory was incorporated into Chinese medicine. The theory holds that "everything in the Universe contains two aspects—*yin* and *yang*, which are in opposition and also in unison. Hence, matters are impelled to develop and change." In traditional Chinese medicine, the phenomena are further explained as follows:

▓ Matters that are dynamic, external, upward, ascending, and brilliant belong to *yang*.

▓ Those that are static, internal, downward, descending, dull, regressive, and hypoactive are *yin*.

▓ *Yin* flourishing and *yang* vivified steadily is the state of health. *Yin* and *yang* regulate themselves in the basic principle to promote the normal activities of life.

▓ Illness is the disharmony of *yin* and *yang*, a disharmony that leads to pathological changes, with excesses of one and deficiencies of the other, disturbances of vital energy and blood, malfunctioning of the viscera, and so forth (Chan 1988).

Table 7-1   **Highlights of Common Elements of Asian Eastern Religions**

The teachings of Asian religions, including Confucianism and Buddhism, are complementary and have played a major role in the shaping of the cultural values in Asia.

Buddhism teaches

- Harmony/nonconfrontation (silence as a virtue)
- Respect for life
- Moderation in behavior, self-discipline, patience, humility, modesty, friendliness, selflessness, dedication, and loyalty to others
- Individualism devalued

Confucianism teaches

- Achievement of harmony through observing the five basic relationships of society
  1. Ruler and ruled
  2. Father and son
  3. Husband and wife
  4. Older and younger brother
  5. Between friends
- Hierarchical roles, social class system, clearly defined behavioral code
- Importance of family
- Filial piety and respect for elders
- High regard for education and learning

Taoism teaches

- Harmony between humans and nature
- Nature is benign because *yin* (evil) and *yang* (good) are in balance and harmony
- Happiness and a long life
- Charity, simplicity, patience, avoidance of confrontation and an indirect approach to problems

Shamanism teaches

- Emphasis on nature
- Everything in nature is endowed with a spirit

Hinduism teaches

- "You can have what you want"
  1. Pleasure—through marriage and family
  2. Success—through vocation
  3. Duty—through civic participation
- The community is greater than ourselves
- The stages of life—student, householder, retirement, and *sannyasin*—"one who neither hates nor loves anything"
- Many paths to the same summit

Source: Romo, R. G. (1995, May 3). Hispanic health traditions and issues. Presented at the Minnesota Health Educators Conference. *Health education expanding our horizons.* Reprinted with permission; Smith, H. (1998). *The world's religions.* New York: HarperCollins.

The various parts of the human body correspond to the dualistic principles of *yin* and *yang*. The inside of the body is *yin*; the surface of the body is *yang*. The front part of the body is *yin*; the back is *yang*. The five *ts'ang* viscera—liver, heart, spleen, lungs, and kidney—are *yang*; the six *fu* structures—gallbladder, stomach, large intestine, small intestine, bladder, and "warmer"—are *yin*. (The "warmer" is now believed to be the lymph system.) The diseases of winter and spring are *yin*; those of summer and fall are *yang*. The pulses are controlled by *yin* and *yang*. If *yin* is too strong, the person is nervous and apprehensive and catches colds easily. If the individual does not balance *yin* and *yang* properly, his or her life will be short. Half of the *yin* forces are depleted by age 40, at 40 the body is sluggish, and at 60 the *yin* is totally depleted, at which time the body deteriorates. *Yin* stores the vital strength of life. *Yang* protects the body from outside forces, and it, too, must be carefully maintained. If *yang* is not cared for, the viscera are thrown into disorder, and circulation ceases. *Yin* and *yang* cannot be injured by evil influences. When *yin* and *yang* are sound, the person lives in peaceful interaction with mind and body in proper order (Wallnöfer & von Rottauscher, 1972).

Chinese medicine has a long history. The Emperor Shen Nung, who died in 2697 B.C., was known as the patron god of agriculture. He was given this title because of the 70 experiments he performed on himself by swallowing a different plant every day and studying the effects. During this period of self-experimentation, Nung discovered many poisonous herbs and rendered them harmless by the use of antidotes, which he also discovered. His patron element was fire, for which he was known as the Red Emperor. The Emperor Shen Nung was followed by Huang-ti, whose patron element was earth. Huang-ti was known as the Yellow Emperor and ruled from 2697 B.C. to 2595 B.C. The greater part of his life was devoted to the study of medicine. Many people ascribe to him the recording of the *Nei Ching*, the book that embraces the entire realm of Chinese medical knowledge. The treatments described in the *Nei Ching*—which became characteristic of Chinese medical practices—are almost totally aimed at reestablishing balances that are lost within the body when ILLNESS occurs. Disrupted harmonies are regarded as the sole cause of disease. Surgery was rarely resorted to; when it was, it was used primarily to remove malignant tumors. The *Nei Ching* is a dialogue between Huang-ti and his minister, Ch'i Po. It begins with the concept of the Tao and the cosmological patterns of the universe and goes on to describe the powers of the *yin* and *yang*. This learned treatise discusses in great detail the therapy of the pulses and how a diagnosis can be made on the basis of alterations in the pulse beat. It also describes various kinds of fevers and the use of acupuncture (Wallnöfer & von Rottauscher, 1972, pp. 26–28).

The Chinese view their bodies as a gift given to them by their parents and forebears. A person's body is not his or her personal property. It must be cared for and well maintained. Confucius taught that "only those shall be truly revered who at the end of their lives will return their physical bodies whole and sound."

The body is composed of five solid organs (*ts'ang*), which collect and store secretions, and five hollow organs (*fu*), which excrete. The heart and liver are regarded as the noble organs. The head is the storage chamber for knowledge, the back is the home of the chest, the loins store the kidneys, the knees store the muscles, and the bones store the marrow.

The Chinese view the functions of the various organs as comparable to the functions of persons in positions of power and responsibility in the government. For example, the heart is the ruler over all other civil servants, the lungs are the administrators, the liver is the general who initiates all the strategic actions, and the gallbladder is the decision maker.

The organs have a complex relationship, which maintains the balance and harmony of the body. Each organ is associated with a color. For example, the heart—which works in accordance with the pulse, controls the kidneys, and harmonizes with bitter flavors—is red. In addition, the organs have what is referred to as an "aura," the meaning of which, in the medical context, is HEALTH. The aura is determined by the color of the organ. In the balanced, healthy body, the colors look fresh and shiny.

Disease is caused by an upset in the balance of *yin* and *yang*. The weather, too, has an effect on the body's balance and the body's relationship to *yin* and *yang*. For example, heat can be injurious to the heart, and cold is injurious to the lungs. Overexertion is harmful to the body. Prolonged sitting is harmful to the flesh and spine, and prolonged lying in bed can be harmful to the lungs.

Disease is diagnosed by the Chinese physician through inspection and palpation. During inspection, the Chinese physician looks at the tongue (glossoscopy), listens and smells (osphretics), and asks questions (anamnesis). During palpation, the physician feels the pulse (sphygmopalpation).

The Chinese believe that there are many different pulse types, which are all grouped together and must be felt with the three middle fingers. The pulse is considered the storehouse of the blood, and a person with a strong, regular pulse is considered to be in good health. By the nature of the pulse, the physician is able to determine various illnesses. For example, if the pulse is weak and skips beats, the person may have a cardiac problem. If the pulse is too strong, the person's body is distended (Wallnöfer & von Rottauscher, 1972).

There are 6 different pulses, three in each hand. Each pulse is specifically related to various organs, and each pulse has its own characteristics. According to ancient Chinese sources, there are 15 ways of characterizing the pulses. Each of these descriptions accurately determines the diagnosis. There are 7 *piao* pulses (superficial) and eight *li* pulses (sunken). An example of an illness that manifests with a *piao* pulse is headache; anxiety manifests with a *li* pulse. The pulses also take on a specific nature with various conditions. For example, specific pulses are associated with epilepsy, pregnancy, and the time just before death.

The Chinese physician is aided in making a diagnosis by the appearance of the patient's tongue. More than 100 conditions can be determined by glossoscopic examination. The color of the tongue and the part of the tongue that does not appear normal are the essential clues to the diagnosis.

Breast cancer has been known to the Chinese since early times. "The disease begins with a knot in the breast, the size of a bean, and gradually swells to the size of an egg. After seven or eight months it perforates. When it has perforated, it is very difficult to cure" (Wallnöfer & von Rottauscher, 1972).

Traditional Methods of HEALTH Maintenance and Protection

There are countless ways by which HEALTH is maintained. One example is the practices involved in daily nutrition. Foods, such as thousand-year eggs, are ingested on a daily basis. There are strict rules governing food combinations and foods that must be eaten preceding and after life events, such as childbirth and surgery. Daily exercise is also important, and many people participate in formal exercise programs, such as tai chi.

The Chinese often prepare amulets to prevent evil spirits and protect HEALTH. These amulets consist of a charm with an idol or a Chinese character painted in red or black ink and written on a strip of yellow paper. These amulets are hung over a door or pasted on a curtain or wall, worn in the hair, or placed in a red bag and pinned on clothing. The paper may be burned and the ashes mixed in hot tea and swallowed to ward off evil. Jade is believed to be the most precious of all stones because it is seen as the giver of children, HEALTH immortality, wisdom, power, victory, growth, and food. Jade charms are worn to bring HEALTH and, should they turn dull or break, the wearer will surely meet misfortune. The charm prevents harm and accidents. Children are kept safe with jade charms, and adults are made pure, just, humane, and intelligent by wearing them (Morgan, 1942 [1972], pp. 133–134).

Traditional Methods of HEALTH Restoration

Just as there are countless methods used to maintain and protect HEALTH, there are countless ways to restore HEALTH. The following discussion describes traditional methods of restoring HEALTH.

Acupuncture

Acupuncture is an ancient Chinese practice of puncturing the body to cure disease or relieve pain. The body is punctured with special metal needles at points that are precisely predetermined for the treatment of specific symptoms. According to one source, the earliest use of this method was recorded between 106 B.C. and A.D. 200. According to other sources, however, it was used even earlier. This treatment modality stems from diagnostic procedures described earlier. The most important aspect of the practice of acupuncture is the acquired skill and ability to know precisely where to puncture the skin. Nine needles are used in acupuncture, each with a specific purpose. The following is a list of the needles and their purposes (Wallnöfer & von Rottauscher, 1972).

- Superficial pricking: arrowhead needle
- Massaging: round needle
- Knocking or pressing: blunt needle
- Venous pricking: sharp three-edged needle
- Evacuating pus: swordlike needle
- Rapid pricking: sharp, round needle

- Puncturing thick muscle: sharp, round needle
- Puncturing thick muscle: long needle
- Treating arthritis: large needle
- Most extensively used: filiform needle

The specific points of the body into which the needles are inserted are known as meridians. Acupuncture is based on the concept that certain meridians extend internally throughout the body in a fixed network. There are 365 points on the skin where these lines emerge. Since all the networks merge and have their outlets on the skin, the way to treat internal problems is to puncture the meridians, which are also categorically identified in terms of *yin* and *yang*, as are the diseases. The treatment goal is to restore the balance of *yin* and *yang* (Wallnöfer & von Rottauscher, 1972). The practice of this art is far too complex to explain in great detail in these pages.

Readers may find it interesting to visit acupuncture clinics in their area. After the therapist carefully explains the art and science of acupuncture, one may be able to grasp the fundamental concepts of this ancient treatment. The practice of acupuncture is based in antiquity, yet it took a long time for it to be accepted as a legitimate method of healing by practitioners of the Western medical system. Currently, numerous acupuncture clinics attract a fair number of non-Asians, and acupuncture is being used as a method of anesthesia in some hospitals.

Moxibustion, Cupping, Bleeding, and Tui Na

Moxibustion has been practiced for as long as acupuncture. Its purpose, too, is to restore the proper balance of *yin* and *yang*. Moxibustion is based on the therapeutic value of heat, whereas acupuncture is a cold treatment. Acupuncture is used mainly in diseases in which there is an excess of *yang*, and moxibustion is used in diseases in which there is an excess of *yin*. Moxibustion is performed by heating pulverized wormwood and passing this concoction above the skin, but not touching it, over certain specific meridians. Great caution must be used in this application because it cannot be applied to all the meridians that are used for acupuncture. Moxibustion is believed to be most useful during the period of labor and delivery, if applied properly.

Other important traditional HEALTH restoring practices are cupping, bleeding, and a form of traditional massage, *Tui Na*.

- Cupping, as seen in Figure 7–1, involves creating a vacuum in a small glass by burning the oxygen out of it, then promptly placing the glass on the person's skin surface. Cupping draws blood and lymph to the body's surface that is under the cup. This increases the local circulation. The purpose for doing this is to remove cold and damp "evils" from the body and/or to assist blood circulation. The procedure is frequently used to treat lung congestion.
- Bleeding, often done with the use of leeches, is performed to "remove heat from the body." Only small amounts of blood are removed.

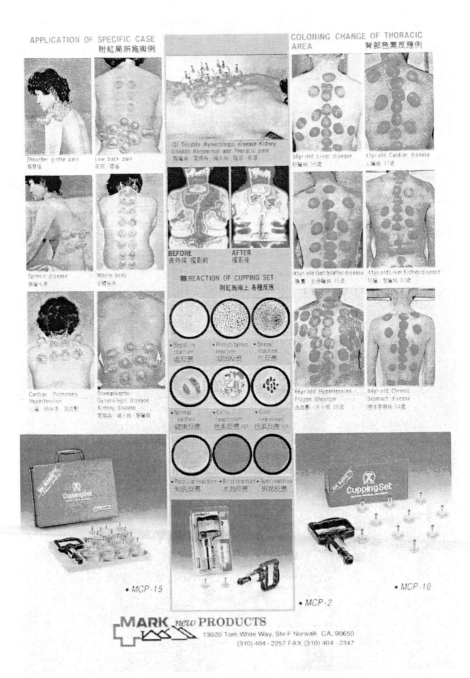

Figure 7-1　Cupping.

■ Massage, *Tui Na*, "pushing and pulling," is a complex system of massage or manual acupuncture point stimulation that is used on orthopedic and neurological conditions (Ergil, 1996, pp. 208–209).

Herbal Remedies

Medicinal herbs were used widely in the practice of ancient Chinese healing. Many of these herbs are available and in use today.

Herbology is an interesting subject. The gathering season of an herb was important for its effect. It was believed that some herbs were better if gathered at night and that others were more effective if gathered at dawn. The ancient sages understood quite well the dynamics of growth. It is known today that a plant may not be effective if the dew has been allowed to dry on its leaves. The herbalist believes that the ginseng root must be harvested only at midnight in a full moon if it is to have therapeutic value. Ginseng's therapeutic value is due to its nonspecific action. The herb, which is derived from the root of a plant that resembles a person, is recommended for use in more than two dozen ailments, including anemia, colics, depression, indigestion, impotence, and rheumatism (Wallnöfer & von Rottauscher, 1972). It has maintained its reputation for centuries and continues to be a highly valued and widely used substance.

To release all the therapeutic properties of ginseng and to prepare it properly are of paramount importance. Ginseng must not be prepared in anything made of metal because it is believed that some of the necessary constituents are leeched out by the action of the metal. It must be stored in crockery. It is boiled in water until only a sediment remains. This sediment is pressed into a crock and stored. Following are some of the specific uses of ginseng (Wallnöfer & von Rottauscher, 1972):

■ To stimulate digestion: rub ginseng to a powder, mix with the white of an egg, and take three times per day.
■ As a sedative: prepare a light broth of ginseng and bamboo leaves.
■ For faintness after childbirth: administer a strong brew of ginseng several times a day.
■ As a restorative for frail children: give a dash of raw, minced ginseng several times per day.

There are many Chinese medicinal herbs, but none is as famous as ginseng.

Step inside a Chinese pharmacy and you will notice drawers containing herbs. Herbs are weighed in the preparation of a prescription. In general, the herbs are wrapped in cheesecloth and placed in a determined amount of boiling water for a determined amount of time. The resulting liquid is then ingested in specific amounts, at specific times each day. The amount of time that the herbs are boiled determines the concentration of the medicine. Thus, the directions for preparation are carefully followed.

The Chinese doctor who practices in the pharmacy writes the prescription, and the cost of filling a prescription varies from nominal ($5.00) to quite expensive (several hundred dollars), depending on the herbs that are used.

In addition to herbs and plants, the Chinese use other products with medicinal and healing properties. Some of these products were also used in ancient Europe and are still used today. For example, in China, boys' urine was used to cure lung diseases, soothe inflamed throats, and dissolve blood clots in pregnant women. In Europe, it was used during the two world wars as emergency treatment for open wounds. Urea is still used today as a treatment that promotes the healing of wounds. Other popular Chinese remedies include

- Deer antlers—used to strengthen bones, increase a man's potency, and dispel nightmares
- Lime calcium—used to clear excessive mucus
- Quicksilver—used externally to treat venereal diseases
- Rhinoceros horns—highly effective when applied to pus boils; an antitoxin for snakebites
- Turtle shells—used to stimulate weak kidneys and to remove gallstones
- Snake flesh—eaten as a delicacy to keep eyes healthy and vision clear
- Seahorses—pulverized and used to treat gout

Traditional HEALERS

The physician was the primary HEALER in Chinese medicine. Physicians who had to treat women encountered numerous difficulties because men were not allowed to touch women directly who were not family members. Thus, a diagnosis might be made through a ribbon that was attached to the woman's wrist. As an alternative to demonstrating areas of pain or discomfort on a woman's body, an alabaster figure was substituted. The area of pain was pointed out on the figurine (Dolan, 1973, p. 30).

Not much is known about women doctors except that they did exist. Women were known to possess a large store of medical talent. There were also midwives and female shamans. The female shamans possessed gifts of prophecy. They danced themselves into ecstatic trances and had a profound effect on the people around them. As the knowledge that these women possessed was neither known nor understood by the general population, they were feared rather than respected. They were said to know all there was to know about life, death, and birth.

Chinese Pediatrics

Babies are generally breast-fed because neither cow's milk nor goat's milk is acceptable to the Chinese. Sometimes children are nursed for as long as 4 or 5 years. However, the practice is now varying as more women are working.

Since early time the Chinese have known about and practiced immunization against smallpox. A child was inoculated with the live virus from the crust of a pustule from a smallpox victim. The crust was ground into a powder, and this powder was subsequently blown into the nose of the healthy child through the lumen of a small tube. If the child was healthy, he or she did not generally develop a full-blown case of smallpox but, instead, acquired immunity to this dreaded disease (Wallnöfer & von Rottauscher, 1972).

Current Health Problems

In many instances, people who were born in the United States into families established here for generations are largely indistinguishable from the general population in their health care beliefs. Other groups, however, especially new immigrants, differ from the general population on many social and health-related issues. In each of the selected categories, the rates for the Asian/Pacific Islander population are lower than those for the general population.

Poor health, however, continues to be found among the residents of Chinatowns partly because of poor working and crowded living conditions. Many people work long hours in restaurants and laundries and receive the lowest possible wages for their hard work. Many cannot afford even minimal, let alone preventive, health care. Americans of Asian and Pacific Island heritage frequently experience unique barriers, including linguistic and cultural differences, when they try to access the unfamiliar health care system.

Language difficulties and adherence to native Chinese culture compound problems already associated with poverty, crowding, and poor health. Many people still prefer the traditional forms of Chinese medicine and seek help from Chinatown "physicians" who treat them with traditional herbs and other methods. Often, Asian people do not seek help from the Western system at all. Others use Chinese methods in conjunction with Western methods of health care, although the Chinese find many aspects of Western medicine distasteful. For example, they cannot understand why so many diagnostic tests, some of which are painful, are necessary. They do, however, accept the practice of immunization and the use of x-rays. An example of a modern health care practice that may cause a problem is the drawing of blood.

Chinese people cannot understand why the often frequent taking of blood samples, considered routine in Western medicine, is necessary. Blood is seen as the source of life for the entire body, and it is believed that blood is not regenerated. The Asian reluctance to have blood drawn for diagnostic tests may have its roots in the revered teachings of Confucius. The Chinese people also believe that a good physician should be able to make a diagnosis simply by examining a person. Consequently, they do not react well to the often painful procedures used in Western diagnostic workups. Some people—because of their distaste for the drawing of blood—leave the Western system rather than tolerate the pain. The Chinese have deep respect for their bodies and believe that it is best to die with their bodies intact. For this reason, many people refuse surgery or consent to it only under the most dire circumstances. This reluctance to undergo intrusive surgical procedures has deep implications for those concerned with providing health care to Asian Americans.

Table 7-2 Comparison of the 10 Leading Causes of Death for Asian/Pacific Islanders American and for All Persons: 2004

Asian/Pacific Islanders American	All Persons
1. Malignant neoplasms	Diseases of heart
2. Diseases of heart	Malignant neoplasms
3. Cerebrovascular diseases	Cerebrovascular diseases
4. Unintentional injuries	Chronic lower respiratory diseases
5. Diabetes mellitus	Unintentional injuries
6. Influenza and pneumonia	Diabetes mellitus
7. Chronic lower respiratory diseases	Alzheimer's disease
8. Suicide	Influenza and pneumonia
9. Nephritis, nephrotic syndrome, and nephrosis	Nephritis, nephrotic syndrome, and nephrosis
10. Alzheimer's disease	Septicemia

Source: National Center for Health Statistics. (2007). *Health, United States, 2007 with chartbook on trends in the health of Americans* (pp.186–187). Hyattsville, MD: Author.

The hospital is an alien place to the Asian people. Not only are the customs and practices strange but also the patients often are isolated from the rest of their people, which enhances the language barrier and feelings of helplessness. Something as basic as food creates another problem. Hospital food is strange to Asian patients and is served in an unfamiliar manner. The typical Chinese patient rarely complains about what bothers him or her. Often the only indication that there may be a problem is an untouched food tray and the silent withdrawal of the patient. Unfortunately, the silence may be regarded by the nurses as reflecting good, complacent behavior, and the health care team exerts little energy to go beyond the assumption. The Chinese patient who says little and complies with all treatment is seen as stoic, and there is little awareness that deep problems may underlie this "exemplary" behavior. Ignorance on the part of health care workers may cause the patient a great deal of suffering.

Much action has been taken in recent years to make Western health care more available and appealing to the Chinese. In Boston, for example, there is a health clinic staffed primarily by Chinese dialects–speaking nurses and physicians who work as paid employees and as volunteers. Most of the common health-related pamphlets have been translated into Chinese languages and into Vietnamese, Cambodian, and Laotian, and they are distributed to the patients. Booklets on such topics as breast self-examination and smoking cessation are available. Since the languages spoken in the clinic are Mandarin Chinese and other dialects, the problem of interpreters has been largely eliminated. The care is personal, and the patients are made to feel comfortable. Unnecessary and painful tests are avoided as much as possible. In addition, the clinic, which is open for long hours, provides social services and employment placements and is quite popular with the community. Although it began as a part-time, storefront operation, the clinic is now housed in its own building.

Table 7–2 compares the 10 leading causes of death among Asian/Pacific Islanders with those of the general population.

The following is a synopsis of cultural beliefs regarding mental health and illness, possible causes of mental illness, and methods of preventing mental illness among people of Asian/Pacific Island origin. Lack of knowledge or skills in mental health therapy is seen in the Asian communities, as mental illness is much ignored in medical classics. Two points must be noted: the importance placed on the family in caring for the mentally ill and the tendency to identify mental illness in somatic terms. There is a tremendous amount of stigma attached to mental illness. Asian patients tend to come to the attention of mental health workers late in the course of their illness, and they come with a feeling of hopelessness (Lin, 1982, pp. 69–73).

One example of cross-cultural therapy is the Japanese practice of Morita therapy. This 70-year-old treatment originated from a treatment for shinkeishitsu, a form of compulsive neurosis with aspects of neurasthenia. The patient is separated from the family for 1 to 2 weeks and taught that one's feelings are the same as the Japanese sky and instantly changeable. One cannot be responsible for how one feels, only for what one does. At the end of therapy, the patient focuses on what is being done and less on his or her inner feelings, symptoms, concerns, or obsessive thoughts (Yamamoto, 1982, p. 50). In addition, there are countless culture-bound mental HEALTH syndromes that may be identified in the Asian communities:

■ Korea—*Hwa-byung*—a syndrome attributed to the suppression of anger is known as "anger syndrome"; symptoms include insomnia, indigestion, and dyspnea

■ China—*Koro*—the occurrence of sudden, intense anxiety when a man believes his penis is folding into his body

■ Japan—*Taijin kyofusho*—intense anxiety about possibly offending others (Fontaine, 2003, p. 119)

Explore ⊕ MediaLink

Go to the Companion Website at www.prenhall.com/spector for chapter-related review questions, case studies, and activities. Contents of the CulturalCare Guide and CulturalCare Museum can also be found on the Companion Website. Click on Chapter 9 to select the activities for this chapter.

Internet Sources

Hay, V. (1994). An Interview with Deepak Chopra. A Magazine of People and Possibilities online http://www.intouchmag.com/chopra.html

National Center for Alternative and Complimentary Medicine. (2007). Backgrounder: What is Ayurvedic Medicine? Bethesda, Maryland: Author. Retrieved July 2, 2007, from http://nccam.nih.gov/health/ayurveda/

Sai Movement. (2002). *Shri SaiBaba of Shirdi* the Perfect Master of the Age. Shirdi, India: *Shri SaiBaba* Trust. Retrieved August 27, 2007 from http://www.shrisaibabasansthan.org/

Somnath, S., and Shipman, S. (2006). The rationale for diversity in the health professions: A review of the evidence (Washington, DC: U.S. Department of Health and Human Services, Health Resources and Services Administration Bureau of Health Professions. http://www.hrsa.gov/

U.S. Census Bureau, Census 2000. Special Tabulations. Profile of Selected Demographic and Social Characteristics: 2000 Asia, China, and India. Retrieved June 9, 2007 from http://factfinder.census.gov, http://www.census.gov/population/cen2000/stp-159/STP-159-Asia.pdf, http://www.census.gov/population/cen2000/stp-159/STP-159-China.pdf, http://www.census.gov/population/cen2000/stp-159/STP-159India.pdf

United States Department of Commerce, U.S. Census Bureau. Census 2000. (2002). Retrieved July 21, 2007 from http://www.census.gov/

United States Department of Health and Human Services, Health Resources and Services. (2004). The National Survey of Registered Nurses 2004 Documentation for the General Public Use File, 2006, Bureau of Health Professions Health Resources and Services Administration. HRSA/BHPr and the National Sample Survey of Registered Nurses. http://www.hrsa.gov/

References

Barnes, J. S., & Bennett, C. E. (2002). *The Asian population: 2000.* Washington, DC: U.S. Department of Commerce.

Chan, P. K. (1988, August 3). Herb specialist, interview by author. New York City. Dr. Chan prepared a supplemental written statement in Chinese and English for inclusion in this text.

Dolan, J. (1973). *Nursing in society: A historical perspective.* Philadelphia: W. B. Saunders. National Center for Health Statistics.

Ergil, K. V. (1996). China's traditional medicine. In M. S. Micozzi (Ed.), *Fundamentals of complementary and alternative medicine,* New York: Churchill Livingstone.

Fontaine, K. L. (2003). *Mental health nursing* (5th ed.). Upper Saddle River, NJ: Prentice Hall.

Fugh-Berman, A. (1996). *Alternative medicine: What works.* Tucson, AZ: Odonian Press.

Grieco, E. M. (2001). *The Native Hawaiian and other Pacific Islander population: 2000.* Washington, DC: U.S. Department of Commerce.

Lin, K. M. (1982). Cultural aspects in mental health for Asian Americans. In A. Gaw (Ed.), *Cross-cultural psychiatry.* Boston: John Wright.

Mann, F. (1972). *Acupuncture.* New York: Vintage Books.

Martin, J. A. (1995). Birth characteristics for Asian or Pacific Islander subgroups, 1992. *Monthly Vital Statistics Report, 43*(10), 1.

Morgan, H. T. (1942 [1972]). *Chinese symbols and superstitions.* Detroit, MI: Gale Research. Reprint, S. Pasadena, CA: Ione Perkins.

National Center for Health Statistics. (2006). *Health, United States, 2006 with chartbook on trends in the health of Americans.* Hyattsville, MD: Author.

National Center for Health Statistics. (2007). *Health, United States, 2007 with chartbook on trends in the health of Americans.* Hyattsville, MD: Author.

Romo, R. G. (1995, May 3). *Hispanic health traditions and issues.* Paper presented at the Minnesota Health Educators Conference.

Roy, C. (1999). *Nurse's handbook of alternative and complementary therapies.* Springhouse, PAS: Springhouse.

Smith, H. (1958). *The religions of man.* New York: Harper & Row.

Spector, R. (1992). Culture, ethnicity, and nursing. In P. Potter & A. Perry (Eds.), *Fundamentals of nursing.* St. Louis: Mosby-Year Book.

U.S. Census Bureau. (2002). *A profile of the nation's foreign-born population from Asia.* Washington, DC: U.S. Department of Commerce.

Wallnöfer, H., & von Rottauscher, A. (1972). *Chinese folk medicine.* M. Palmedo (Trans.), New York: American Library.

Yamamoto, J. (1982). Japanese Americans. In A. Gaw (Ed.), *Cross-cultural psychiatry.* Boston: John Wright.

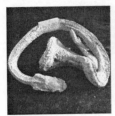 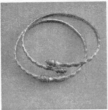 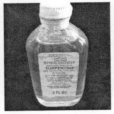 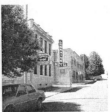

Chapter 8

HEALTH and ILLNESS in the Black Population

Who are we? We are the embodiment of the American dream, the architects of rock and roll, the builders of the cities, and the artisans on the assembly line. We are deep and real.

—*Bass & Pugh (2001)*

■ Objectives

1. Discuss the background of members of the Black population.
2. Describe the traditional definitions of *HEALTH* and *ILLNESS* of members of the Black population.
3. Describe the traditional methods of HEALTH maintenance and protection of selected communities of the Black population.
4. Describe current health care problems of members of the Black population.

The opening photos depict HEALTH-related items that may be used by people of Black, or African American, heritage to protect, maintain, and/or restore their HEALTH. The dried garden snake is ground up and brewed as a tea, and the liquid may be used to treat skin blemishes. Silver bangle bracelets from Saint Thomas, the Virgin Islands, are open to let out evil yet closed to prevent evil from entering the body. They are said to tarnish when the person wearing them is vulnerable to ILLNESS; this alerts the person to take better care of him- or herself. They are worn from birth, and many people believe that they will die if they remove them. Often, many bracelets are worn together, and the bell-like sound that they make when they touch is said to scare the evil spirits away. These are worn to protect HEALTH. Rectified turpentine with sugar is used to treat a cough. Nine drops of turpentine 9 days after intercourse may act as a contraceptive. Sugar and turpentine may also be used to get rid of intestinal worms. The last segment is the Lorraine Hotel in Memphis, Tennessee, the site of the assassination of Dr. Martin Luther King, Jr., in 1968.

▓ Background

"Black or African American" refers to people having origins in any of the Black race groups of Africa (McKinnon, 2001, p. 1). Blacks or African Americans are the largest emerging majority population in the United States, constituting an estimated 12.3% of the U.S. population in 2000 (Dalaku, 2001, p. 1) and 12.8% of the U.S. population of the United States in 2005.

"Black" is used in this chapter's text to refer to the Black or African American population, but "Black or African American" is used in tables and figures. This follows the pattern used in Census 2000. Most members of the present Black American community have their roots in Africa, and the majority descend from people who were brought here as slaves from the west coast of Africa (Bullough & Bullough, 1972, pp. 39–41). The largest importation of slaves occurred during the 17th century, which means that Black people have been living in the United States for many generations. Today, a number of Blacks have immigrated to the United States voluntarily—from African countries, the West Indian islands, the Dominican Republic, Haiti, and Jamaica.

Black Americans live in all regions of the country. In 2000, the majority of the Black population, 54.8%, lived in the South. About three fifths of all people who reported their racial identity as Black lived in the following 10 states: New York (3.2 million), California (2.5 million), Texas (2.5 million), Florida (2.5 million), Georgia (2.4 million), Illinois, North Carolina, Maryland, Michigan, and Louisiana. The cities with the largest numbers of Blacks were New York, Chicago, Detroit, Memphis, and Houston.

Blacks are represented in every socioeconomic group; however, 22.1% of the group lived in poverty in 2000 and in 2005 the percentage was 24.9. Blacks have remained disproportionately poor (Dalaku, 2001, p. 1). Furthermore, over half of Black Americans live in urban areas surrounded by the symptoms of poverty—crowded and inadequate housing, poor schools, and high crime rates.

For example, Kotlowitz (1991) described the Henry Horner Homes in Chicago as "16 high-rise buildings which stretch over eight blocks and at last census count housed 6,000 people, 4,000 of whom are children." The degree of social and economic change between 1990 and 2000 has been minimal. He presented two facts about public housing: "Public housing served as a bulwark to segregation and as a kind of anchor for impoverished neighborhoods" and "It was built on the cheap—the walls are a naked cinder block with heating pipes snaking through the apartment; instead of closets, there are eight-inch indentations in the walls without doors; and the heating system so storms out of control in the winter that it is 85 degrees." Situations similar to this prevail presently. The Black population is also young, 54.5% of the Black population in combination with one or more races are under 18 (Dalaku, 2001, p. 9), and the mean age in 2005 was 32.4 years.

There are now a growing number of people arriving from Africa as new immigrants. The total population of people born in Africa and who have entered the United States since before 1980 and 2000 is 881,300; from Nigeria 134,940; from Somalia 36,760; and from Sudan 19,790 (U.S. Census Bureau). The rates of naturalization, learning English, and educational achievement are low as of this writing.

According to some sources, the first Black people to enter this country arrived a year earlier than the Pilgrims, in 1619. Other sources claim that Blacks arrived with Columbus in the 15th century (Bullough & Bullough, 1972, pp. 39–41). In any event, the first Blacks who came to the North American continent did not come as slaves, but, between 1619 and 1860, more than 4 million people were transported here as slaves. One need read only a sampling of the many accounts of slavery to appreciate the tremendous hardships that the captured and enslaved people experienced during that time. Not only was the daily life of the slave very difficult, but the experience of being captured, shackled, and transported in steerage was devastating. Many of those captured in Africa died before they arrived here. The strongest and healthiest people were snatched from their homes by slave dealers and transported en masse in the holds of ships to the North American continent. In general, Black captives were not taken care of or recognized as human beings and treated accordingly. Once here, they were sold and placed on plantations and in homes all over the country—it was only later that the practice was confined to the South. Families were separated; children were wrenched from their parents and sold to other buyers. Some slave owners bred their slaves much as farmers breed cattle today, purchasing men to serve as studs, and judging women based on whether they would produce the desired stock with a particular man (Haley, 1976). However, in the midst of all this inhuman and inhumane treatment, the Black family grew and survived. Gutman (1976), in his careful documentation of plantation and family records, traces the history of the Black family from 1750 to 1925 and points out the existence of families and family or kinship ties before and after the Civil War, dispelling many of the myths about the Black family and its structure. Despite overwhelming hardships and enforced separations, the people managed in most circumstances to maintain both a family and community awareness.

The people who came to America from West Africa brought a rich variety of traditional beliefs and practices and came from religious traditions that respected the spiritual power of ancestors. They worshiped a diverse pantheon of gods, who oversaw all aspects of daily life, such as the changes of the seasons, the fertility of nature, physical and spiritual personal health, and communal success. Initiation rites and naming rituals, folktales, and healing practices, dance, song, and drumming were a part of the religious heritage. Many aspects of today's Christian religious practices are believed to have originated in these practices. In addition, it has been estimated that between 10% and 30% of the slaves brought to America between 1711 and 1808 were Muslim. The people brought their prayer practices, fasting and dietary practices, and their knowledge of the Qur'an (Eck, 1994).

Ostensibly, the Civil War ended slavery, but in many ways it did not emancipate Blacks. Daily life after the war was fraught with tremendous difficulty, and Black people—according to custom—were stripped of their civil rights. In the South, Black people were overtly segregated, most living in conditions of extreme hardship and poverty. Those who migrated to the North over the years were subject to all the problems of fragmented urban life: poverty, racism, and covert segregation (Bullough & Bullough, 1972, p. 43; Kain, 1969, pp. 1–30).

The historic problems of the Black community need to be appreciated by the health care provider who attempts to juxtapose modern practices and traditional health and illness beliefs. In addition, health care providers must be aware of the ongoing and historical events in the struggle for civil rights that affect people's lives. In 2007 the Supreme Court ruled in *Parents v. Seattle Schools* and *Meredith v. Jefferson Schools* that public schools can't consider race when making student school assignments. This may be viewed as an effort to strike down *Brown v. Board of Education*, the landmark ruling of 1956. Also, in 2007, James Ford Seale, a Mississippi Klansman was sentenced to three life terms in prison for the Moore/Dee murder of 1964.

■ Traditional Definitions of *HEALTH* and *ILLNESS*

According to Jacques (1976), the traditional definition of *HEALTH* stems from the African belief about life and the nature of being. To the African, life was a process rather than a state. The nature of a person was viewed in terms of energy force rather than matter. All things, whether living or dead, were believed to influence one another. Therefore, one had the power to influence one's destiny and that of others through the use of behavior, whether proper or otherwise, as well as through knowledge of the person and the world. When one possessed HEALTH, one was in harmony with nature; ILLNESS was a state of disharmony. Traditional Black belief regarding HEALTH did not separate the mind, body, and spirit.

Disharmony—that is, ILLNESS—was attributed to a number of sources, primarily demons and evil spirits. These spirits were generally believed to act of their own accord, and the goal of treatment was to remove them from the body of the ILL person. Several methods were employed to attain this result, in addition to voodoo, which is discussed in the next section. The traditional healers, usually women, possessed extensive knowledge of the use of herbs and roots in the treatment of ILLNESS. Apparently, an early form of smallpox immunization was used by slaves. Women practiced inoculation by scraping a piece of cowpox crust into a place on a child's arm. These children appeared to have a far lower incidence of smallpox than those who did not receive the immunization.

The old and the young were cared for by all members of the community. The elderly were held in high esteem because African people believed that the living of a long life indicated that a person had the opportunity to acquire much wisdom and knowledge. Death was described as the passing from one realm of life to another (Jacques, 1976, p. 117) or as a passage from the evils of this world to another state. The funeral was often celebrated as a joyous occasion, with a party after the burial. Children were passed over the body of the deceased, so that the dead person could carry any potential illness of the child away with him or her.

Many of the preventive and treatment practices of Black people have their roots in Africa but have been merged with the approaches of Native Americans, to whom the Blacks were exposed, and with the attitudes of Whites among whom they lived and served. Then, as today, ILLNESS was treated in a combination of ways. Methods found to be most useful were handed down through the generations.

■ Traditional Methods of HEALTH Maintenance and Protection

The following sections present examples of practices employed presently or in earlier generations to maintain and protect HEALTH and to treat various types of maladies to restore HEALTH. This discussion cannot encompass all the types of care given to and by the members of the Black community but instead presents a sample of the richness of the traditional HEALTH practices that have survived over the years.

Essentially, HEALTH is maintained with proper diet—that is, eating three nutritious meals a day, including a hot breakfast. Rest and a clean environment also are important. Laxatives were and are used to keep the system "running" or "open."

Asafetida—rotten flesh that looks like a dried-out sponge—is worn around the neck to prevent the contraction of contagious diseases. Cod liver oil is taken to prevent colds. A sulfur and molasses preparation is used in the spring because it is believed that at the start of a new season people are more susceptible to illness. This preparation is rubbed up and down the back, not taken internally. A physician is not consulted routinely and is not generally regarded as the person to whom one goes for the prevention of disease.

Copper or silver bracelets may be worn around the wrist from the time a woman is a baby or young child. These bracelets are believed to protect the wearer as she grows. If for any reason these bracelets are removed, harm befalls the owner. In addition to granting protection, these bracelets indicate when the wearer is about to become ill: the skin around the bracelet turns black, alerting the woman to take precautions against the impending illness. These precautions consist of getting extra rest, praying more frequently, and eating a more nutritious diet.

Traditional Methods of HEALTH Restoration

The most common method of treating ILLNESS is prayer. The laying on of hands is described quite frequently. Rooting, a practice derived from voodoo, also is mentioned by many people. In rooting, a person (usually a woman who is known as a "root-worker)" is consulted as to the source of a given ILLNESS, and she then prescribes the appropriate treatment. Magic rituals often are employed (Davis, 1998).

The following home remedies have been reported by some Black people as being successful in the treatment of disease.

1. Sugar and turpentine are mixed together and taken by mouth to get rid of worms. This combination can also be used to cure a backache when rubbed on the skin from the navel to the back.

2. Numerous types of poultices are employed to fight infection and inflammation. The poultices are placed on the part of the body that is painful or infected to draw out the cause of the affliction. One type of poultice is made of potatoes. The potatoes are sliced or grated and placed in a bag, which is placed on the affected area of the body. The potatoes turn black; as this occurs, the disease goes away. It is believed that, as these potatoes spoil, they produce a penicillin mold that is able to destroy the infectious organism. Another type of poultice is prepared from cornmeal and peach leaves, which are cooked together and placed either in a bag or in a piece of flannel cloth. The cornmeal ferments and combines with an enzyme in the peach leaves to produce an antiseptic that destroys the bacteria and hastens the healing process. A third poultice, made with onions, is used to heal infections, and a flaxseed poultice is used to treat earaches.

3. Herbs from the woods are used in many ways. Herb teas are prepared—for example, from goldenrod root—to treat pain and reduce fevers. Sassafrass tea frequently is used to treat colds. Another herb boiled to make a tea is the root or leaf of rabbit tobacco.

4. Bluestone, a mineral found in the ground, is used as medicine for open wounds. The stone is crushed into a powder and sprinkled on the affected area. It prevents inflammation and is used to treat poison ivy.

5. To treat a "crick" in the neck, two pieces of silverware are crossed over the painful area in the form of an X.

6. Nine drops of turpentine 9 days after intercourse act as a contraceptive.

7. Cuts and wounds can be treated with sour or spoiled milk that is placed on stale bread, wrapped in a cloth, and placed on the wound.

8. Salt and pork (salt pork) placed on a rag can be used to treat cuts and wounds.

9. A sprained ankle can be treated by placing clay in a dark leaf and wrapping it around the ankle.

10. A remedy for treating colds is hot lemon water with honey.

11. When congestion is present in the chest and the person is coughing, the chest is rubbed with hot camphorated oil and wrapped with warm flannel.

12. An expectorant for colds consists of chopped raw garlic, chopped onion, fresh parsley, and a little water, all mixed in a blender.

13. Hot toddies are used to treat colds and congestion. These drinks consist of hot tea with honey, lemon, peppermint, and a dash of brandy or whatever alcoholic beverage the person likes and is available. Vicks Vaporub also is swallowed.

14. A fever can be broken by placing raw onions on the feet and wrapping the feet in warm blankets.

15. Boils are treated by cracking a raw egg, peeling the white skin off the inside of the shell, and placing it on the boil. This brings the boil to a head.

16. Garlic can be placed on the ill person or in the room to remove the "evil spirits" that have caused the illness.

Folk Medicine

In the Black community, folk medicine previously practiced in Africa is still employed. The methods have been tried and tested and are still relied on. Healers or voodoo practitioners make no class or status distinctions among their patients, treating everyone fairly and honestly. This tradition of equality of care and perceived effectiveness accounts for the faith placed in the practices of the HEALER and in other methods. In fact, the home remedies used by some members of the Black community have been employed for many generations. Another reason for their ongoing use is that hospitals are distant from people who live in rural areas. By the time they might get to the hospital, they would be dead, yet many of the people who continue to use these remedies live in urban areas close to hospitals—sometimes even world-renowned hospitals. Nonetheless, the use of folk medicine persists, and many people avoid the local hospital except in extreme emergencies.

▨ Current Health Problems

Health Differences between Black and White Populations

Morbidity. Many people experience factors such as the lack of access to health services, low income, and a tendency to self-treat illness and to wait until symptoms are so severe that a doctor must be seen. When statistical adjustments are made for age, Blacks exceed Whites in the average number of days spent in acute care settings, on bed rest, and in restricted activity. In addition, Blacks have a greater incidence of tooth decay and periodontal disease than Whites (National Center for Health Statistics, 2006, pp. 278, 279). Adolescent pregnancy is a major concern with the population. The risk of infant mortality and low birth weight are also greater in the community, as is the rate of low-birth-weight babies.

Sickle-Cell Anemia. The sickling of red blood cells is a genetically inherited trait that is hypothesized to have originally been an African adaptation to fight malaria. This condition occurs only in Blacks and causes the normal, disk-like red blood cell to assume a sickle shape. Sickling results in hemolysis and thrombosis of red blood cells because these deformed cells do not flow properly through the blood vessels.

Some people (carriers) have the sickle-cell trait (HbSS, HbSC, or others) but do not experience symptoms of the disease.

The clinical manifestations of sickle-cell disease include hemolysis, anemia, and states of sickle-cell crises, in which severe pain occurs in the areas of the body where the thrombosed red cells are located. The cells also tend to clump in abdominal organs, such as the liver and the spleen. At present, statistics indicate that only 50% of children with sickle-cell disease live to adulthood. Some children die before the age of 20, and some suffer chronic, irreversible complications during their lifetime.

It is possible to detect the sickle-cell trait in healthy adults and to provide genetic counseling about their risk of bearing children with the disease. However, for many people, this is not an option (Bullock & Jilly, 1975, pp. 234–272). The cost of genetic counseling, for example, may be prohibitive.

Mortality. Blacks born in 2000 in the United States will live, on average, 5.7 fewer years than Whites. The life expectancy for Whites born in 2000 is 77.6 years; for Blacks, it is 71.9 years (National Center for Health Statistics, 2007, p. 175).

The leading chronic diseases that are causes of death for African Americans are the same as those for Whites, but the rates are greater:

- Blacks die from strokes at almost twice the rate of the White population. (National Center for Health Statistics, 2007, p. 204).
- Coronary heart disease death rates are higher for Blacks than for Whites.
- Black men experience a higher risk of cancer of the prostate than White men do.
- Homicide is the most frequent cause of death for Black American men between the ages of 25 and 34 the rate in 2004 was 81.6 per 100,000 resident population. (NCHS, 2007, p. 227)
- The rate of AIDS among Black American men generally is higher than that for White men and the mortality rate for both Black men, 29.2/100,000 and women, 13.0/100,000 resident population in 2004 is the highest rate. (NCHS, p. 219)

Mental Health Traditions

The family often has a matriarchal structure, and there are many single-parent households headed by females but there are strong and large extended family networks. There are a continuation of tradition and a strong church affiliation within the families and community. Members of the community may be treated by a traditional voodoo priest, the "Old Lady" ("granny" or "Mrs. Markus"), or other traditional healers, and herbs are frequently used to treat mental symptoms. Several diagnostic techniques include the use of biblical phrases and/or material from old folk medical books, observation, and/or entering the spirit of the patient. The therapeutic measures include various rituals, such as the reading of bones, the wearing of special garments, or some rituals from voodoo (Spurlock, 1988, p. 173).

Blacks and the Health Care System

To some, receiving health care is all too often a degrading and humiliating experience. In many settings, Black patients continue to be viewed as beneath the White health care giver. Quite often, the insult is a subtle part of experiencing the health care system. The insult may be intentional or unintentional. An intentional insult is, of course, a blatant remark or mistreatment. An unintentional insult is more difficult to define. A health care provider may not intend to demean a person, yet an action or a tone of voice may be interpreted as insulting. The provider may have some covert, underlying fears or difficulties in relating to Blacks, but the patient quite often senses the difficulty. An unintentional insult may occur because the provider is not fully aware of the patient's background and is unable to comprehend many of the patient's beliefs and practices. The patient, for example, may be afraid of the impending medical procedures and the possibility of misdiagnosis or mistreatment. It is not a secret among the people of the Black community that those who receive care in public clinics and hospitals—and even in clinics of private institutions—are the "material" on whom students practice and on whom medical research is done.

Some Blacks fear or resent health clinics. When they have a clinic appointment, they usually lose a day's work because they have to be at the clinic at an early hour and often spend many hours waiting to be seen by a physician. They often receive inadequate care, are told what their problem is in incomprehensible medical jargon, and are not given an identity, being seen rather as a body segment ("the appendix in treatment room A"). Such an experience creates a tremendous feeling of powerlessness and alienation from the system. In some parts of the country, segregation and racism are overt. There continue to be reports of hospitals that refuse admission to Black patients. In one case, a Black woman in labor was not admitted to a hospital because she had not "paid the bill from the last baby." There was not enough time to get her to another hospital, and she was forced to deliver in an ambulance. In light of this type of treatment, it is no wonder that some Black people prefer to use time-tested home remedies rather than be exposed to the humiliating experiences of hospitalization.

Another reason for the ongoing use of home remedies is poverty. Indigent people cannot afford the high costs of American health care. Quite often—even with the help of Medicaid and Medicare—the hidden costs of acquiring health services, such as absence from work, transportation, and/or child care, are a heavy burden. As a result, Blacks may stay away from clinics or outpatient departments or receive their care with passivity while appearing to the provider to be evasive. Some Black patients believe that they are being talked down to by health care providers and that the providers fail to listen to them. They choose, consequently, to "suffer in silence." Many of the problems that Blacks relate in dealing with the health care system can apply to anyone, but the inherent racism within the health system cannot be denied. Currently, efforts are being made to overcome these barriers.

Since the 1960s, health care services available to Blacks and other people of color have improved. A growing number of community health centers have emphasized health maintenance and promotion. Community residents serve on the boards.

Among the services provided by community health centers is an effort to discover children with high blood levels of lead in order to provide early diagnosis of and treatment for lead poisoning. Once a child is found to have lead poisoning, the law requires that the source of the lead be found and eradicated. Today, only apartments free of lead paint can be rented to families with young children. Apartments that are found to have lead paint must be stripped and repainted with nonlead paint. Another ongoing effort by the community health centers is to inform Blacks who are at risk of producing children with sickle-cell anemia that they are carriers of this genetic disease. This program is fraught with conflict because many people prefer not to be screened for the sickle-cell trait, fearing they may become labeled once the tendency is discovered.

Birth control is another problem that is recognized with mixed emotions. To some, especially women who want to space children or who do not want to have numerous children, birth control is a welcome development. People who believe in birth control prefer selecting the time when they will have children, how many children they will have, and when they will stop having children. To many other people, birth control is considered a form of "Black genocide" and a way of limiting the growth of the community. Health workers in the Black community must be aware of both sides of this issue and, if asked to make a decision, remain neutral. Such decisions must be made by the patients themselves.

Special Considerations for Health Care Providers

White health care providers know far too little about how to care for a Black person's skin or hair, or how to understand both Black nonverbal and verbal behavior.

Physiological Assessment. Examples of possible physiological problems include the following (in observing skin problems, it is important to note that skin assessment is best done in indirect sunlight) (Bloch & Hunter, 1981):

1. **Pallor.** There is an absence of underlying red tones; the skin of a brown-skinned person appears yellow-brown, and that of a black-skinned person appears ashen gray. Mucous membranes appear ashen, and the lips and nailbeds are similar.

2. **Erythema.** Inflammation must be detected by palpation; the skin is warmer in the area, tight, and edematous, and the deeper tissues are hard. Fingertips must be used for this assessment, as with rashes, since they are sensitive to the feeling of different textures of skin.

3. **Cyanosis.** Cyanosis is difficult to observe in dark-colored skin, but it can be seen by close inspection of the lips, tongue, conjunctiva, palms of the hands, and soles of the feet. One method of testing is pressing the palms. Slow blood return is an indication of cyanosis. Another sign is ashen gray lips and tongue.

4. **Ecchymosis.** History of trauma to a given area can be detected from a swelling of the skin surface.

5. **Jaundice.** The sclera are usually observed for yellow discoloration to reveal jaundice. This is not always a valid indication, however, since carotene deposits can also cause the sclera to appear yellow. The buccal mucosa and the palms of the hands and soles of the feet may appear yellow.

Several skin conditions are of importance in Black patients (Sykes & Kelly, 1979):

1. **Keloids.** Keloids are scars that form at the site of a wound and grow beyond the normal boundaries of the wound. They are sharply elevated and irregular and continue to enlarge.

2. **Pigmentary disorders.** Pigmentary disorders, areas of either postinflammatory hypopigmentation or hyperpigmentation, appear as dark or light spots.

3. **Pseudofolliculitis.** "Razor bumps" and "ingrown hairs" are caused by shaving too closely with an electric razor or straight razor. The sharp point of the hair, if shaved too close, enters the skin and induces an immune response as to a foreign body. The symptoms include papules, pustules, and sometimes even keloids.

4. **Melasma.** The "mask of pregnancy," melasma, is a patchy tan to dark brown discoloration of the face more prevalent in dark pregnant women.

Explore 🌐 MediaLink

Go to the Companion Website at www.prenhall.com/spector for chapter-related review questions, case studies, and activities. Contents of the CulturalCare Guide and CulturalCare Museum can also be found on the Companion Website. Click on Chapter 10 to select the activities for this chapter.

Internet Sources

Brunner, B., and Haney, E. (2007). Civil Rights Timeline: Milestones in the modern civil rights movement. Upper Saddle River, NJ: Pearson Education. Retrieved June 9, 2007 from http://www.infoplease.com/spot/civilrightstimeline1.html

Hogan, H., and Lamas, E. J. (2007). The American Community—Blacks: 2004. Washington, D.C.: U. S. Census Bureau. Retrieved from http://www.census.gov/population/www/socdemo/race.html, February 24, 2008

Ibrahim, I. A. (2002). A Brief Illustrated Guide to Understanding Islam. Houston, Texas: Darussalam. Retrieved from http://www.islam-guide.com/frm-editors.htm, July 21, 2007.

Office of Dawah. (2006–2008). The Religion of Islam. Rawdah: Author. Retrieved Sept. 19, 2007 from http://www.islamreligion.com/

Somnath, S., and Shipman, S. (2006). The rationale for diversity in the health professions: A review of the evidence (Washington, DC: U.S. Department of Health and Human Services, Health Resources and Services Administration Bureau of Health Professions. http://www.hrsa.gov/, January 5, 2008

United States Census Bureau, Census 2000 Special Tabulations. Profile of Selected Demographic and Social Characteristics: 2000 Africa, Nigeria, Somalia, and Sudan. Retrieved July 25, 2007 from http://www.census.gov/population/cen2000/stp-159/STP-159-Africaica.pdf, http://www.census.gov/population/cen2000/stp-159/STP-159-Nigeria.pdf, http://www.census.gov/population/cen2000/stp-159/STP-159-Somalia.pdf, and http://www.census.gov/population/cen2000/stp-159/STP-159-Sudan.pdf

United States Department of Health and Human Services. (2004). The Registered Nurse Population Findings from the March, 2004 National Sample of Registered Nurses. Washington DC: Author. Retrieved from ftp://ftp.hrsa.gov/bhpr/workforce/0306rnss.pdf, January 5, 2008

References

American Psychiatric Association. (1994). *Diagnostic and statistical manual of mental disorders* (4th ed.). Washington, DC: Author.

Bass, P. H., & Pugh, K. (2001). *In our own image—Treasured African-American traditions, journeys, and icons.* Philadelphia: Running Press.

Bloch, B., & Hunter, M. L. (1981, January–February). Teaching physiological assessment of Black persons. *Nurse Educator*, 26.

Bullock, W. H., & Jilly, P. N. (1975). Hematology. In R. A. Williams (Ed.), *Textbook of Black-related diseases.* New York: McGraw-Hill.

Bullough, B., & Bullough, V. L. (1972). *Poverty, ethnic identity, and health care.* New York: Appleton-Century-Crofts.

Dalaku, J. (2001). *Poverty in the United States: 2000.* U.S. Census Bureau Current Population Reports Series P60-214. Washington, DC: U.S. Government Printing Office.

Davis, R. (1998). *American voudou—Journey into a hidden world.* Denton: University of North Texas Press.

Dunstin, B. (1969). Pica during pregnancy. Chap. 26 in *Current concepts in clinical nursing.* St. Louis, MO: Mosby.

Eck, D. (1994). *African religion in America: On common ground.* New York: Columbia University Press.

Fontaine, K. L. (2003). *Mental health nursing* (5th ed.). Upper Saddle River, NJ: Prentice Hall.

Gutman, H. G. (1976). *The Black family in slavery and freedom, 1750–1925.* New York: Pantheon.

Haley, A. (1976). *Roots.* New York: Doubleday.

Hughes, L., & Bontemps, A. (Eds.), (1958). *The book of negro folklore.* New York: Dodd, Mead.

Jacques, G. (1976). Cultural health traditions: A Black perspective. In M. Branch & P. P. Paxton (Eds.), *Providing safe nursing care for ethnic people of color.* New York: Appleton-Century-Crofts.

Kain, J. F. (Ed.). (1969). *Race and poverty.* Englewood Cliffs, NJ: Prentice Hall.

Kotlowitz, A. (1991). *There are no children here: The story of two boys growing up in the other America.* New York: Doubleday.

Manderschied, R. W., & Sonnenschein, M. A. (Eds.). (1992). *Mental health, United States.* Washington, DC: Center for Mental Health Services and National Institute of Mental Health, DHHS Pub. No. (SMA) 92-1942, U.S. Government Printing Office.

McKinnon, J. (2001). *The Black population: 2000.* Washington, DC: U.S. Census Bureau.

National Center for Health Statistics. (2006). *Health, United States, 2006 with chartbook on trends in the health of Americans.* Hyattsville, MD: Author.

National Center for Health Statistics. (2007). *Health, United States, 2007 with chartbook on trends in the health of Americans.* Hyattsville, MD: Author.

Spector, R. (1992). Culture, ethnicity, and nursing. In P. Potter & A. Perry (Eds.), *Fundamentals of nursing* (3rd ed.). St. Louis: Mosby-Year Book.

Spurlock, J. (1988). Black Americans. In L. Comas-Diaz & E. E. H. Griffith (Eds.), *Cross-cultural mental health.* New York: John Wiley & Sons.

Sykes, J., & Kelly, A. P. (1979, June). Black skin problems. *American Journal of Nursing,* 1092–1094.

Tallant, R. (1946). *Voodoo in New Orleans* (7th printing). New York: Collier.

Webb, J. Y. (1971). Letter. Dr. J. R. Krevans to Y. Webb, 15 February 1967. Reported in *Superstitious influence—VooDoo in particular—Affecting health practices in a selected population in southern Louisiana.* Paper. New Orleans, LA.

Wintrob, R. (1972). Hexes, roots, snake eggs? M.D. vs. occults. *Medical Opinion, 1*(7), 54–61.

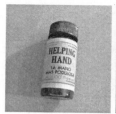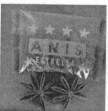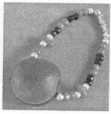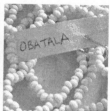

Chapter 9

HEALTH and ILLNESS in the Hispanic Populations

My heart is in the earth . . .

—*Greenhaw (2000)*

▓ Objectives

1. Discuss the background of members of selected communities of the Hispanic populations.
2. Describe the traditional definitions of *HEALTH* and *ILLNESS* of selected communities of the Hispanic populations.
3. Describe the traditional methods of HEALTH maintenance and protection of selected communities of the Hispanic populations.
4. Describe the traditional methods of HEALING of selected communities of the Hispanic populations.
5. Describe current health care problems of the Hispanic populations.

The images opening this chapter are examples of the many remedies and objects a person may purchase to protect, maintain, and/or restore HEALTH. The first item is "helping hand oil"; it is applied to the body to protect the wearer from *mal ojo*, the evil eye. The second item is anise, licorice, a popular herbal remedy that is prepared as a tea and used to soothe the stomach. The third item is a "deer's eye" bracelet for a baby or child; it is used to ward off the evil eye and bring good luck. The last item represents the beads of *Santeria*. These beads are worn by a person whose patron, or *Orisha*, is *Obatala*. *Obatala* is the major Yoruba deity and father of the Yoruba gods. The discussion later in this chapter will provide an explanation of the *Orishas*, or gods of *Santeria*.

▓ Background

The largest emerging majority group in the United States is composed of the Hispanic or Latino populations. The terms *Hispanic* and *Latino* are used inter-changeably in Census 2000 and will be used accordingly in this chapter. This is done to reflect the new terminology in the standards issued by the Office of Management and Budget in 1997, used in the reporting of Census 2000, and became official in 2003 (Therrien & Ramirez, 2001, p. 1). The term *Hispanic,* or *Latino, Americans* refers to people who were born in or whose predecessors came from (even generations ago) Mexico, Puerto Rico, Cuba, Central and South America, Spain, and other Spanish-speaking communities and who now live in the United States. The Hispanic people constituted 9% of the population in the 1990 census, grew to 12% in 2000, and reached 15% in 2005. They are the fastest growing and, with a mean age of 25.8 years and a median age of 24 years, the youngest population group.

The most recent analysis of demographic data, 2002, relevant to the Hispanic community showed

- ▓ Hispanics are more geographically concentrated than non-Hispanic Whites, with 44.2% living in the West and 34.8% living in the South.
- ▓ Hispanics are more likely than non-Hispanic Whites to be less than 18 years old, as 34.4% of Hispanics are younger than 5 and 22.8% of the non-Hispanic White population are younger than 5.
- ▓ Two in five Hispanics are foreign-born.
- ▓ Hispanics live in family households that are larger than those of non-Hispanic Whites.
- ▓ The percentage of Hispanics graduating from high school or attending some college was 45.9% in 2002 and having at least a high school diploma was 45.9% in 2002, as compared to non-Hispanic Whites, for whom the percentages were 59.3% graduating from high school or attending some college and 88.7% having at least a high school diploma.
- ▓ Hispanics were much more likely than non-Hispanic Whites to not have full-time year-round employment with annual earnings of $35,000 or more in 2001.

■ Hispanics were more likely than non-Hispanic Whites to live in poverty—21.4% of the Hispanic population and 7.8% of the White alone population. (Ramirez & de la Cruz, 2003, pp. 1–6)

There have been 16,089,975 people legally admitted from Latin America; with 480,665 people from Guatemala, and 9,177,485 people from Mexico. The percentages of people who have been naturalized as citizens are low and one factor that is reported by community workers is money. In fact, the fee to apply for citizenship rose from $400 to $675 on July 30, 2007 (Ballou, 2007, p. B5).

Mexicans

The United States shares a 2,000-mile-long border with Mexico, which, in spite of walls and tightened security, remains easily crossed in both directions. The flow of people, goods, and ideas across it has a powerful impact on both countries.

Americans of Hispanic origin, according to the 2002 census, numbered at least 37.4 million people; of this number, 66.9% were of Mexican origin (Ramirez & de la Cruz, 2002, p. 1). The Mexicans have been in the United States for a long time, moving from Mexico and later intermarrying with Indians and Spanish people in the southwestern parts of what is now the United States. Santa Fe, New Mexico was settled in 1609. Most of the descendants of these early settlers now live in Arizona, California, Colorado, New Mexico, and Texas. A large number of Mexicans also live in Illinois, Indiana, Kansas, Michigan, Missouri, Nebraska, New York, Ohio, Utah, Washington, and Wisconsin, where most arrived as migrant farm workers. While located there as temporary farm workers, they found permanent jobs and stayed. Contrary to the popular views that Mexicans live in rural areas, most live in urban areas. Mexicans are employed in all types of jobs. Few, however, have high-paying or high-status jobs in labor or management. The majority work in factories, mines, and construction; others are employed in farm work and service areas. At present, only a small—though growing—number are employed in clerical and professional areas. The number of unemployed in this group is high (estimated to be between 25% and 30%), and the earnings of those employed are well below the national average. The education of Mexicans, like that of most minorities in the United States, lags behind that of most of the population. Many Mexicans fail to complete high school. In the past few years, this situation has begun to change, and Mexican children are being encouraged to stay in school, go on to college, and enter the professions.

Traditional Definitions of HEALTH and ILLNESS

There are conflicting reports about the traditional meaning of HEALTH among Mexicans. Some sources maintain that HEALTH is considered to be purely the result of "good luck" and that a person loses his or her health if that luck changes (Welch, Comer, & Steinman, 1973, p. 205). Some people describe HEALTH as a reward for good behavior. Seen in this context, HEALTH is a gift from God and should not be taken for granted. People are expected to maintain their own equilibrium in the universe by performing in the proper way, eating the proper foods, and working the proper amount of time. The protection of HEALTH is an accepted practice that is accomplished with prayer, the wearing of religious medals or amulets, and the keeping of relics in the home. Herbs and spices can be used to enhance this form of prevention, as can exemplary behavior (Lucero, 1975). ILLNESS is seen as an imbalance in an individual's body or as punishment meted out for wrongdoing. The causes of ILLNESS can be grouped into five major categories:

1. *The body's imbalance.* Imbalance may exist between "hot" and "cold" or "wet" and "dry." The theory of hot and cold was taken to Mexico by Spanish priests and was fused with Aztec beliefs. The concept actually dates to the early Hippocratic theory of disease and four body humors. The disrupted relationship among these humors is often mentioned by Mexicans as the cause of disease (Lucero, 1975).

   There are four body humors, or fluids: (1) blood, hot and wet; (2) yellow bile, hot and dry; (3) phlegm, cold and wet; and (4) black bile, cold and dry. When all four humors are balanced, the body is HEALTHY. When any imbalance occurs, an ILLNESS is manifested (Currier, 1966). These concepts, of course, provide one way of determining the remedy for a particular ILLNESS. For example, if an ILLNESS is classified as hot, it is treated with a cold substance. A cold disease, in turn, must be treated with a hot substance. Food, beverages, animals, and people possess the characteristics of hot and cold to various degrees. Hot foods cannot be combined; they are to be eaten with cold foods. There is no general agreement as to what is a hot disease or food and what is a cold disease or food. The classification varies from person to person, and what is hot to one person may be cold to another (Saunders, 1958, p. 13). Therefore, if a Mexican patient refuses to eat the meals in the hospital, it is wise to ask precisely what the person can eat and what combinations of foods he or she thinks would be helpful for the existing condition. It is important to note that *hot* and *cold* do not refer to temperature but are descriptive of a particular substance itself.

   For example, after a woman delivers a baby, a hot experience, she cannot eat pork, which is considered a hot food. She must eat something cold to restore her balance. Penicillin is a hot medication; therefore, it may be believed that it cannot be used to treat a hot disease. The major problem for the health care provider is to know that the rules, so to speak, of hot and cold vary from person to person. If health care providers understand the general nature of the hot and cold imbalance, they will be able to help the patient reveal the nature of the problem from the patient's perspective and manage it accordingly.

2. *Dislocation of parts of the body.* Two examples of "dislocation" are *empacho* and *caida de la mollera* (Nall & Spielberg, 1967). *Empacho* is believed to be caused by a ball of food clinging to the wall of the stomach. Common symptoms of this illness are stomach pains and cramps. This ailment is treated by rubbing and gently pinching the spine. Prayers are recited throughout the treatment. Another, more common, cause of such illness is thought to be lying about the amount of food consumed. A 20-year-old Hispanic woman experienced the acute onset of sharp abdominal pain. She complained to her friend, and together they diagnosed the problem as *empacho* and treated it by massaging her stomach and waiting for the pain to dissipate. It did not, and they continued folk treatment for 48 hours. When the pain did not diminish, they sought help in a nearby hospital. The diagnosis was acute appendicitis. The young woman nearly died and was quite embarrassed when she was scolded by the physician for not seeking help sooner.

   Caida de la mollera is a more serious illness. It occurs in infants and young children aged under 1 year who are dehydrated (usually because of diarrhea or severe vomiting) and whose anterior fontanelle is depressed below the contour of the skull (Dorsey & Jackson, 1976, p. 56). Much superstition and mystery surround this problem. Some of the poorly educated and rural people, in particular, may believe that it is caused by a nurse's or physician's having touched the baby's head. This can be understood if we take into account that (1) an infant's fontanelle becomes depressed if the infant is dehydrated and (2) when physicians or nurses measure an infant's head they touch this area. If a mother takes her baby to a physician for an examination and sees the physician touch the child's head, and if the baby gets sick thereafter with *caida de la mollera,* it might be very easy for the woman to believe it is the fault of the physician's or nurse's touch. Unfortunately, epidemics of diarrhea are common in the rural and urban areas of the Southwest, and a number of children tend to be affected. One case of severe dehydration that leads to *caida de la mollera* may create quite a stir among the people. The folk treatment of this illness has not been found to be effective. Unfortunately, babies are rarely taken to the hospital in time, and the mortality rate for this illness is high (Lucero, 1975).

3. *Magic or supernatural causes outside the body.* Witchcraft or possession is considered to be culturally patterned role-playing, a safe vehicle for restoring oneself. Witchcraft or possession legitimizes acting out bizarre behavior or engaging in incoherent speech. Hispanic tradition, especially in the Borderlands (the geographic area along the United States/Mexico border) blends the medieval heritage of medieval Castilian and English traditions with Mexican Indian folk beliefs (Kearney & Medrano, 2001, p. 119). *Brujas* (witches) use black, or malevolent, magic, while *curanderos* use white, or benevolent,

magic. Spells may be cast to influence a lover or to get back at a rival, and cards are read to tell the future. *Herbrias* sell herbs, amulets, and talismans (Kearney & Medrano, p. 117).

A lesser disease that is caused from outside the body is *mal ojo*. *Mal ojo* means "bad eye," and it is believed to result from excessive admiration on the part of another. General malaise, sleepiness, fatigue, and severe headache are the symptoms of this condition. The folk treatment is to find the person who has caused the illness by casting the "bad eye" and having him or her care for the afflicted person (Nall & Spielberg, 1967). The belief in the evil eye, *mal de ojo*, can be traced back to the mid-1400s and Spain (Kearney & Medrano, 2001, p. 118). It has origins that go back even further in many parts of the world. This belief is common today.

4. *Strong emotional states. Susto* is described as an illness arising from fright. It afflicts many people—males and females, rich and poor, rural dwellers and urbanites. It involves soul loss: The soul is able to leave the body and wander freely. This can occur while a person is dreaming or when a person experiences a particularly traumatic event. The symptoms of the disease are (1) restlessness while sleeping; (2) listlessness, anorexia, and disinterest in personal appearance when awake, including disinterest in both clothing and personal hygiene; and (3) loss of strength, depression, and introversion. The person is treated by *curandero* (a folk healer, discussed above and in the section on *curanderismo*), who coaxes the soul back into the person's body. During the healing rites, the person is massaged and made to relax (Rubel, 1964).

5. *Envidia. Envidia,* or envy, also is considered to be a cause of illness and bad luck. Many people believe that to succeed is to fail. That is, when one's success provokes the envy of friends and neighbors, misfortune can befall the person and his or her family. For example, a successful farmer, just when he is able to purchase extra clothing and equipment, is stricken with a fatal illness. He may well attribute the cause of this illness to the envy of his peers. A number of social scientists have, after much research, concluded that the "low" economic and success rates of Mexicans can ostensibly be attributed to belief in *envidia* (Lucero, 1975).

Curanderismo

There are no specific rules for knowing who in the community uses the services of folk healers. Not all Mexicans do, and not all Mexicans believe in their precepts. Initially, it was thought that only the poor used a folk healer, or *curandero*, because they were unable to get treatment from the larger, institutionalized health care establishments. It now appears, however, that the use of HEALERS occurs widely throughout the Mexican population. Some people try to use HEALERS exclusively, whereas others use them along with institutionalized care. The HEALERS do not usually advertise, but they are well known throughout the population because of informal community and kinship networks.

Curanderismo is defined as a medical system (Maduro, 1976). It is a coherent view with historical roots that combine Aztec, Spanish, spiritualistic, homeopathic, and scientific elements. There are curanderos practicing in Spain, and there is an established community of curanderos in close proximity to Granada.

The curandero(a) is a holistic healer. The people who seek help from him or her do so for social, physical, and psychological purposes. The curandero(a) can be either a "specialist" or a "generalist," a full-time or part-time practitioner. Mexicans who believe in curanderos consider them to be religious figures.

A curandero(a) may receive the "gift of healing" through three means:

1. He or she may be "born" to heal. In this case, it is known from the moment of a cuandero(a)'s birth that something unique about this person means that he or she is destined to be a healer.
2. He or she may learn by apprenticeship—that is, the person is taught the ways of healing, especially the use of herbs.
3. He or she may receive a "calling" through a dream, trance, or vision by which contact is made with the supernatural by means of a "patron" (or "caller"), who may be a saint. The "call" comes either during adolescence or during the midlife crisis. This "call" is resisted at first. Later, the person becomes resigned to his or her fate and gives in to the demands of the "calling."

HEALTH Restoration

The most popular form of HEALTH restoration used by folk healers involves herbs, especially when used as teas. The curandero knows what specific herbs to use for a problem. This information is revealed in dreams, in which the "patron" gives suggestions.

Because the curandero has a religious orientation, much of the treatment includes elements of both the Catholic and Pentecostal rituals and artifacts: offerings of money, penance, confession, the lighting of candles, milagros, and the laying on of hands. Massage is used in illnesses such as empacho.

Cleanings, the removal of negative forces or spirits, or limpias, are done in two ways. The first is by passing an unbroken egg over the body of the ILL person. The second method entails passing herbs tied in a bunch over the body. The back of the neck, which is considered a vulnerable spot, is given particular attention.

In contrast to the depersonalized care Mexicans expect to receive in medical institutions, their relationship with and care by the curandero are uniquely personal. This special relationship between Mexicans and the curanderos may well account for folk healers' popularity. In addition to the close, personal relationship between patient and healer, other factors may explain the continuing belief in *curanderismo:*

1. The mind and body are inseparable.
2. The central problem of life is to maintain harmony, including social, physical, and psychological aspects of the person.
3. There must be harmony between the hot and cold, wet and dry. The treatment of ILLNESS should restore the body's harmony, which has been lost.
4. The patient is the passive recipient of disease when the disease is caused by an external force. This external force disrupts the natural order of the internal person, and the treatment must be designed to restore this order. The causes of disharmony are evil and witches.
5. A person is related to the spirit world. When the body and soul are separated, soul loss can occur. This loss is sometimes caused by *susto,* a disease or illness resulting from fright, which may afflict individuals from all socioeconomic levels and lifestyles.
6. The responsibility for recovery is shared by the ILL person, the family, and the *curandero(a).*
7. The natural world is not clearly distinguished from the supernatural world. Thus, the *curandero(a)* can coerce, curse, and appease the spirits. The *curandero(a)* places more emphasis on his or her connections with the sacred and the gift of healing than on personal properties. (Such personal properties might include social status, a large home, and expensive material goods.)

Several types of emotional illnesses are found among the traditional people from Hispanic communities. These are further divided into **mental illness** (in which the illness is not judged) and **moral illness** (in which others can judge the victim). The causes of mental illness and examples of the illness they cause are as follows:

■ Heredity—epilepsy (*epilepsia*)
■ Hex—evil eye (*mal ojo*)
■ Worry—anxiety (*tirisia*)
■ Fright—hysteria (*histeria*)
■ Blow to the head—craziness (*locura*)

The causes of moral illness and examples of the illness they cause are as follows:

■ Vice—use of drugs (*drogadicto*)
■ Character weakness—alcoholism (*alcoholismo*)
■ Emotions—jealousy (*celos*) and/or rage (*coraje*) (Spencer, Nichols, Lipkin, et al., 1993, p. 133)

Ethnopharmacologic teas may be used to treat these maladies and amulets may be worn or religious rituals followed to prevent or treat them. The following are examples of herbs that may be purchased in grocery stores, markets, and *botanicas* and are used as teas to treat the listed maladies:

- Camomile tea, *Manzanilla*, used to cure fright
- Spearmint tea, *Yerba Buena*, used to treat nervousness
- Orange leaves, *Te de naranja*, used as a sedative to treat nervousness
- Sweet basil, *Albacar*, used to treat fright and to ward off evil spirits (p. 133)

The HEALTH beliefs and practices discussed here are prevalent today (2008). I recently spoke with an immigrant from a small village in Mexico and inquired about *curanderismo*. He was excited to know that I was familiar with the practice and was proud to share his knowledge and experiences.

Puerto Ricans

Puerto Rican migrants to the United States mainland are American citizens, albeit with a different language and culture. They are neither immigrants nor aliens. According to the 2000 census, 9% of the Hispanic population are Puerto Ricans. Most live on the East Coast, with the greatest number living in New York City and metropolitan New Jersey. Most Puerto Ricans migrate to search for a better life or because relatives, particularly spouses and parents, have migrated previously. Life on the island of Puerto Rico is difficult because there is a high level of unemployment. Puerto Ricans are not well known or understood by the majority of people in the continental United States. Little is known about their cultural identity. Mainlanders tend to forget that Puerto Rico is, for the most part, a poor island whose people have many problems. When many Puerto Ricans migrate to the mainland, they bring many of their problems—especially those with poor health and social circumstance (Cohen, 1972).

Puerto Ricans, along with Cubans, constitute the most recent major immigration group to these shores. They cover the spectrum of racial differences and have practiced racial intermarriage. Many are Catholic, but some belong to Protestant sects.

Many people from Puerto Rico perceive HEALTH and ILLNESS and use folk healers and remedies in ways similar to those used by other Hispanics, whereas others practice *santeria*. Most studies on health and illness beliefs and healing have been conducted on Mexicans. It is not easy to find information about the beliefs of Puerto Ricans. Much of the information presented here was gleaned from students and patients. Both groups feel that their beliefs should be known by health care deliverers. One student, whose mother is a healer and is teaching her daughter the art, corroborated much of the following material.

Common Folk Diseases and Their Treatment

Table 9–1 lists a number of folk diseases and the usual source and type of treatment as reported to me by several Puerto Ricans. Many of these diseases or disharmonies were mentioned in the section on Mexican approaches. Nonetheless, there are subtle differences in the ways folk diseases are perceived by Mexicans and Puerto Ricans. For example, although diseases are classified as hot and cold, treatments—that is, food and medications—are categorized as hot (*caliente*), cold (*frío*), and cool (*fresco*). Cold illnesses are treated with hot remedies; hot diseases are treated with cold or cool remedies. Table 9–2 lists the major illnesses, foods, and medicines and herbs associated with the hot-cold system as it is applied among Puerto Ricans in the United States.

A number of activities are carried out to maintain the proper hot-cold balance in the body.

Examples are as follows:

1. *Pasmo*, a form of paralysis, usually is caused by an upset in the hot-cold balance. For example, if a woman is ironing (hot) and then steps out into the rain (cold), she may get facial or other paralysis.
2. A person who is hot cannot sit under a mango tree (cold) because he or she can get a kidney infection or "back problems."

Table 9–1   Folk Diseases

Name	Description	Treatment	Source of Treatment
Susto	Sudden fright, causing shock	Relaxation	Relative or friend
Fatigue	Asthmalike symptoms	Oxygen; medications	Western health care system
Pasmo	Paralysis-like symptoms, face or limbs	Prevention; massage	Folk
Empacho	Food forms into a ball and clings to the stomach, causing pain and cramps	Strong massage over the stomach; medication; gently pinching and rubbing the spine	Folk
Mal ojo	Sudden, unexplained illness in a usually well child or person	Prevention; babies wear a special charm	Depends on the severity of the symptoms: usually home or folk
Ataque	Screaming; falling to ground; wildly moving arms and legs; hysterical crying	None—ends spontaneously	

3. A baby should not be fed a formula (hot), as it may cause rashes; whole milk (cold) is acceptable.
4. A man who has been working (hot) must not go into the coffee fields (cold), or he could contract a respiratory illness.
5. A hot person must not drink cold water, as it could cause colic.

There is often a considerable time lag between disregarding these precautions and the occurrence of illness. A patient who had injured himself while lifting heavy cartons in a factory revealed that the "true" reason he was now experiencing prolonged back problems was because as a child he often sat under a mango tree when he was "hot" after running. This childhood habit had significantly damaged his back, so that, as an adult, he was unable to lift heavy objects without causing injury. Table 9–2 provides additional examples of this phenomenon.

Table 9-2   The Hot-Cold Classification Among Puerto Ricans

	Frio (Cold)	*Fresco* (Cool)	*Caliente* (Hot)
Illness or bodily conditions	Arthritis Menstrual period Joint pains	Colds	Constipation Diarrhea Pregnancy Rashes Ulcers
Medicine and herbs		Bicarbonate of soda Linden flowers Milk of magnesia Nightshade Orange flower water Sage Tobacco	Anise Aspirin Castor oil Cinnamon Cod-liver oil Iron tablets Penicillin Vitamins
Foods	Avocado Banana Coconut Lima beans Sugar cane White beans	Barley water Whole milk Chicken Fruits Honey Raisins Salt cod Watercress Onions Peas	Alcoholic beverages Chili peppers Chocolate Coffee Corn meal Evaporated milk Garlic Kidney beans

Source: Schilling, B., & Brannon, E. (1986, September). Health-related dietary practices, in *Cross-cultural counseling—A guide for nutrition and health counselors* (p. 5). Alexandra, VA: U.S. Department of Agriculture, U.S. Department of Health and Human Services. Nutrition and Technical Services Division. Reprinted with permission.

The following are examples of selected behaviors a patient may manifest with an illness thought to be caused by an imbalance of hot and cold:

- During pregnancy a woman may avoid hot-classified foods and medicines and take cool-classified medicines.
- During the postpartum period or during menstruation a woman may avoid cool-classified foods and medicines.
- Infant formulas containing evaporated milk, which are hot-classified, may be avoided as the baby is fed cold-classified whole milk.
- Penicillin, a hot-classified prescription, may not be taken for diarrhea, constipation, or a rash, as these are hot-classified symptoms.
- When a diuretic is prescribed that needs to be supplemented with cold-classified bananas or raisins, the bananas or raisins may not be eaten when the disease is a cold-classified condition.

These examples illustrate the use of foods or medicines to restore a sense of balance (Harwood, 1971).

Puerto Ricans also share with others of Hispanic origin a number of beliefs in spirits and spiritualism. They believe that mental illness is caused primarily by evil spirits and forces. People with such disorders are preferably treated by a "spiritualist medium" (Cohen, 1972). The psychiatric clinic is known as the place where locos, mentally ill people, go. This attitude is exemplified in the Puerto Rican approach to visions and the like. The social and cultural environment encourages the acceptance of having visions and hearing voices. In the dominant culture of the continental United States, when one has visions or hears voices, one is encouraged to see a psychiatrist. When a Puerto Rican regards this experience as a problem, he or she may seek help through *Santeria* (Mumford, 1973).

Santeria is the form of Latin American magic that had its birth in Nigeria, the country of origin of the Yoruba people, who were brought to the New World as slaves over 400 years ago. The *Santeria*, or *santero*, may use storytelling as a way of helping people cope with day-to-day difficulties (Flores-Pena, 1991). They brought with them their traditional religion, which was in time synthesized with Catholic images. The believers continue to worship in the traditional way, especially in Puerto Rico, Cuba, and Brazil. The Yorubas identified their gods—*Orishas*—with the Christian saints and invested in these saints the same supernatural powers of gods.

Santeria is a structured system consisting of *espiritismo* (spiritualism), which is practiced by gypsies and mediums who claim to have *facultades* (sacred abilities). These special *facultades* provide them with the "license" to practice. The status or positions of the practitioners form a hierarchy: The head is the *babalow*, a male; second is the *presidente*, the head medium; and third are the *santeros*. Novices are the "believers." The *facultades* are given to the healer from protective Catholic saints, who have African names and are known as *protecciones*. *Santeria* can be practiced in storefronts, basements, homes, and even college dormitories. *Santeros* dress in white robes for ceremonies and wear special beaded bracelets as a sign of their identity.

Puerto Ricans are able to accept much of what Anglos may judge to be idiosyncratic behavior. In fact, behavioral disturbances are seen as symptoms of illness that are to be treated, not judged. Puerto Ricans make a sharp distinction between "nervous" behavior and being *loco*. To be *loco* is to be bad, dangerous, evil. It also means losing all one's social status. Puerto Ricans who seek standard American treatment for mental illness are castigated by the community. They understandably prefer to get help for the symptoms of mental illness from the *santero*, who accepts the symptoms and attributes the cause of the illness to spirits outside the body. Puerto Ricans have great faith in this system of care and maintain a high level of hope for recovery.

The *santero* is an important person, respecting the patient and not gossiping about either the patient or his or her problems. Anyone can pour his or her heart out with no worry of being labeled or judged. The *santero* is able to tell a person what the problem is, prescribe the proper treatment, and tell the person what to do, how to do it, and when to do it. A study in New York found that 73% of the Puerto Rican patients in an outpatient mental health clinic reported having visited a *santero*. Often, a sick person is taken to a psychiatrist by his or her family to be "calmed down" and prepared for treatment by a *santero*. Families may become angry if the psychiatrist does not encourage belief in God and prayer during work with the patient. Because of cultural differences and beliefs, a psychiatrist may diagnose as illness what Puerto Ricans may define as health. Frequently, a spiritualist treats the "mental illness" of a patient as *facultades*, which makes the patient a "special person." Thus, esteem is granted to the patient as a form of treatment. I visited a *santero* in Los Angeles with the hope of his granting me an interview. Instead, he argued that if I wanted to know about his practice I should "sit," so I did. He proceeded to examine my head and palms, throw and read cowerie shells, tell me a story, and asked me to interpret it. Once this was accomplished, he recommended certain interventions. His manner was extremely calming and, when he interpreted the story with me, I discovered his uncanny ability to read habits and behavior (Flores-Pena, 1991). A number of cultural phenomena affect the health and health care of Hispanic Americans (Mumford, 1973).

Current Health Problems

The Hispanic health profile is marked by diversity, and people of the Hispanic community experience perhaps the most varied set of health issues encountered by any of the emerging majority populations. The diversity in health problems is intertwined with the effects of socioeconomic status, as well as with geographic and cultural differences. The most important health issues for Hispanics are related to these demographic facts: The population is young and has a high birth rate.

Hispanics experience a number of barriers when seeking health care. The most obvious one is language. In spite of the fact that Spanish-speaking people constitute one of the largest minority groups in this country, very few health care deliverers speak Spanish. This is especially true in communities in which the number of Spanish-speaking people is relatively small. Hispanics who live in these areas experience tremendous frustration because of the language barrier. Even in large cities, there are far too many occasions when a sick person has to rely on a young child to act not only as a translator but also as an interpreter. One way of sensitizing young nursing students to the pain of this situation is to ask them to present a health problem to a person who does not speak or understand a word of English. Needless to say, this is extremely difficult; it is also embarrassing. People who try this rapidly comprehend and appreciate the feelings of patients who are unable to speak or understand English. (After this experience, two of my students decided to take a foreign-language elective.) Language will continue to be a problem until (1) there are more physicians, nurses, and social workers from the Spanish-speaking communities and (2) more of the present deliverers of health care learn to speak Spanish.

A second crucial barrier that Hispanic people encounter is poverty. The diseases of the poor—for example, tuberculosis, malnutrition, and lead poisoning—all have high incidences among Spanish-speaking populations.

A final barrier to adequate health care is the time orientation of Hispanic Americans. To Hispanics, time is a relative phenomenon. Little attention is given to the exact time of day. The frame of reference is wider, and the issue is whether it is day or night. The American health care system, on the other hand, places great emphasis on promptness. Health care providers demand that clients arrive at the exact time of the appointment—despite the fact that clients are often kept waiting. Health system workers stress the client's promptness rather than their own. In fact, they tend to deny responsibility for the waiting periods by blaming them on the "system." Many facilities commonly schedule all appointments for 9:00 A.M. when it is clearly known and understood by the staff members that the doctor will not even arrive until 11:00 A.M. or later. The Hispanic person frequently responds to this practice by arriving late for appointments or failing to go at all. They prefer to attend walk-in clinics, where the waits are shorter. They also much prefer going to traditional healers.

Explore 🌐 MediaLink

Go to the Companion Website at www.prenhall.com/spector for chapter-related review questions, case studies, and activities. Contents of the CulturalCare Guide and CulturalCare Museum can also be found on the Companion Website. Click on Chapter 11 to select the activities for this chapter.

■ Internet Sources

Grieco, E., and Cassidy, R. C. (2001). Overview of Race and Hispanic Origin. Census Brief. Washington, DC: Census Bureau. Retrieved from http://www.census.gov/prod/2001pubs/c2kbr01-1.pdf July 25, 2007

Ramirez, R., and de la Cruz, G. P. (2002). *The Hispanic population in the United States:* March 2002, Current Population Reports, P20–54, U.S. Census Bureau, Washington, D.C. Retrieved July 25, 2007 from http://www.census.gov/prod/2003pubs/p20–545.pdf.

Somnath, S., and Shipman, S. (2006). The rationale for diversity in the health professions: A review of the evidence (Washington, DC: U.S. Department of Health and Human Services, Health Resources and Services Administration Bureau of Health Professions. http://www.hrsa.gov/ January 5, 2008

U.S. Census Bureau, Census 2000 Special Tabulations. Profile of Selected Demographic and Social Characteristics: 2000 Latin America, Guatemala, Mexico. Retrieved July 25, 2007 from http://www.census.gov/population/cen2000/stp-159/STP-159-LatinAmerica.pdf, http://www.census.gov/population/cen2000/stp-159/STP-159-Guatemala.pdf, and http://www.census.gov/population/cen2000/stp-159/STP-159-Mexico.pdf

United States Department of Health and Human Services. (2004). The Registered Nurse Population Findings from the March, 2004 National Sample of Registered Nurses. Washington DC: Author. Retrieved from ftp://ftp.hrsa.gov/bhpr/workforce/0306rnss.pdf, January 5, 2008

References

Ballou, B. (2007, July 22). *Boston Sunday Globe*, p. B-5.

Carmack, R. M., Gasco, J., & Gossen, G. H. (1996). *The legacy of Mesoamerica.* Upper Saddle River, NJ: Prentice Hall.

Cohen, R. E. (1972, June). Principles of preventive mental health programs for ethnic minority populations: The acculturation of Puerto Ricans to the United States. *American Journal of Psychiatry, 128*(12), 79.

Currier, R. L. (1966, March). The hot-cold syndrome and symbolic balance in Mexican and Spanish-American folk medicine. *Ethnology, 5,* 251–263.

Dorsey, P. R., & Jackson, H. Q. (1976). Cultural health traditions: The Latino/Mexican perspective. In M. F. Branch & P. P. Paxton (Eds.), *Providing safe nursing care for ethnic people of color.* New York: Appleton-Century-Crofts.

Egan, M. (1991). *Milagros.* Santa Fe: Museum of New Mexico Press.

Flores-Pena, Y. & Evanchuk, R. J. (1994). *Santeria garments and alters.* Jackson: University of Mississippi Press.

Flores-Pena, Y. (1991). Personal interview. Los Angeles, CA.

Gonzalez-Wippler, M. (1987). *Santeria—African magic in Latin America.* New York: Original.

Greenhaw, W. (2000). *My heart is in the earth.* Montgomery, AL: River City.

Harwood, A. (1971). The hot-cold theory of disease: Implications for treatment of Puerto Rican patients. *Journal of the American Medical Association, 216,* 1154–1155.

Kearney, M., & Medrano, M. (2001). *Medieval culture and the Mexican American borderlands.* College Station: Texas A & M University Press.

Lucero, G. (1975, March). *Health and illness in the Mexican community.* Lecture given at Boston College School of Nursing.

Maduro, R. J. (1976, January). *Curanderismo: Latin American folk healing.* Conference, San Francisco.

Mumford, E. (1973, November–December). Puerto Rican perspectives on mental illness. *Mount Sinai Journal of Medicine, 40*(6), 771–773.

Nall, F. C., II, & Spielberg, J. (1967). Social and cultural factors in the responses of Mexican-Americans to medical treatment. *Journal of Health and Social Behavior, 8,* 302.

National Center for Health Statistics. (2001). *Health, United States, 2001, with urban and rural health chartbook.* Hyattville, MD: Author.

National Center for Health Statistics. (2006). *Health, United States, 2006 with chartbook on trends in the health of Americans.* Hyattville, MD: Author.

National Center for Health Statistics. (2007). *Health, United States, 2007 with chartbook on trends in the health of Americans.* Hyattville, MD: Author.

Ochoa, C. (December 15, 2007). Personal Telephone Interview. Mission, Texas.

Riva, A. (1990). *Devotions to the saints.* Los Angeles: International Imports.

Rubel, A. J. (1964, July). The epidemiology of a folk illness: Susto in Hispanic America. *Ethnology, 3*(3), 270–271.

Saunders, L. (1958). Healing ways in the Spanish southwest. In E. G., Jaco (Ed.), *Patients, physicians, and illness.* Glencoe, IL: Free Press.

Schilling, B., & Brannon, E. (1986). Health-related dietary practices. In *Cross-cultural counseling: A guide for nutrition and health counselors.* Alexandria, VA: U.S. Department of Health and Human Services.

Spector, R. (1996). *Cultural diversity in health and illness* (4th ed.). Stamford, CT: Appleton & Lange.

Spencer, R. T., Nichols, L. W., Lipkin, G. B., et al. (1993). *Clinical pharmacology and nursing management* (4th ed.). Philadelphia: Lippincott.

Therrien, M., & Ramirez, R. R. (2001). *Hispanic population in the United States, 2000.* Washington, DC: U.S. Census Bureau.

Welch, S., Comer, J., & Steinman, M. (1973, September). Some social and attitudinal correlates of health care among Mexican Americans. *Journal of Health and Social Behavior, 14,* 205.

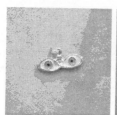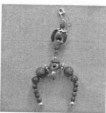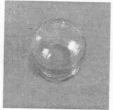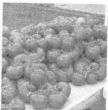

Chapter 10

HEALTH and ILLNESS in the White Populations

Grand Contested Election for the Presidency of the United States.
BLOODY BATTLE IN AFGHANISTAN

—*H. Melville,* Moby Dick *(1851)*

■ Objectives

1. Discuss the background of the White populations.
2. Describe the traditional definitions of *HEALTH* and *ILLNESS* of the White populations.
3. Describe the traditional methods of HEALTH maintenance and protection of selected communities of the White populations.
4. Describe the traditional methods of HEALING of the White populations.
5. Describe health problems of the White populations.

The opening images for this chapter are symbolic of traditional health-related objects that people of White European heritage may use to protect, maintain, and/or restore their HEALTH. The eyes represent the eyes of Saint Lucy, the patron saint of eye diseases and are worn to prevent blindness. The bead and horseshoe, from Armenia, may be pinned on a baby or child for protection from the evil eye. *Bankes*, from Russia and other Eastern European countries, are small, bulb-shaped, thick-glass jars that may be used to create negative pressure to break the congestion that occurs with bronchitis or pneumonia. (*Directions:* Place cotton saturated with alcohol in the jar and light it. Place grease on the skin in the area where you will place the jar. Turn the jar upside down on the skin. The flame goes out. Leave it for 5 minutes and then gently remove the jar. Go to bed and keep warm for several hours.) The *bankes* were commonly used a generation ago and is still used in many places today. The succulent tomatoes are reminders of the nutritional adage to eat "fresh foods" common among Italian gardeners—here is a selection of the early autumn harvest.

■ Background

Members of White European American communities have been immigrating to this country since the very first settlers came to the shores of New England. The White population has diverse and multiple origins. The recent literature in the area of ethnicity and health/HEALTH has focused on people of color, and little has been written about the HEALTH traditions of the White ethnic communities. In this chapter, an overview of the differences in traditional HEALTH beliefs and practices, by ethnicity, is presented. Given that we are talking about 68% of the American population, the enormity of the task of attempting to describe each difference is readily apparent. Instead, this chapter presents an overview of the relevant demographics of the White population, highlights some of the basic beliefs of selected groups (those groups with which I have had the greatest exposure), and presents a comparison of the health status of Whites to the whole population as well as the census cohorts. The overview includes not only library research but also firsthand interviews and observations of people in their daily experiences with the health care delivery system, both as inpatients and as community residents receiving home care.

The major groups migrating to this country between 1820 and 1990 included people from Germany, Italy, the United Kingdom, Ireland, Austria-Hungary, Canada, and Russia; this was a majority of the total immigrant population. However, in 1970, the numbers of immigrants from Europe began to decrease and in 2003 the percentage of foreign-born people from Europe was 13.7% (Larsen, 2004). Chapter 2 explores immigration in greater detail. The 1980 census was the first to include a question about ancestry. The U.S. Census Bureau uses the term **ancestry** to refer to a person's ethnic origin or descent, roots, heritage, or the place of birth of the person or the person's parents or ancestors before their arrival in the United States. Some ethnic identities, such as "German" can be traced to geographic areas outside the United States, while other ethnicities, such as "Pennsylvania Dutch" or "Cajun," evolved in the United States.

The responses to the question of ancestry were a reflection of the ethnic group(s) with which persons identified, and they were able to indicate their ethnic group regardless of how many generations they were removed from it. The following list shows the most common European ancestries in the U.S. population in 2000 (Brittingham, A., and de la Cruz, G. P., 2004 p. 3).

Ancestry	Numbers Identifying Themselves as This Ancestry (Millions)	Percent
German	42.8	15.2
Irish	30.5	10.8
English	24.5	8.7
Italian	15.6	5.6
Polish	9.0	3.2
French (except Basque)	8.3	3.0
Scottish	4.9	1.7

There have been 4,915,555 people admitted from Europe; 706,705 from Germany, 473,340 from Italy, and 466,740 Poland.

The discussion in Chapter 2 referred to age in general; in this chapter, it is important to examine the age of the White populations more specifically. The median age of Whites alone is 38 years, the oldest of each population group. In addition, it is important to note that the percentage of people over 65 in the total population is 12.4, whereas for Whites alone the number is 14.4%, and the percentage of the total population under 18 is 25.7% and for Whites alone it is 23.5% (Meyer, 2001, p. 5).

An additional facet to note is that in many cities the White alone population is now a minority. These cities include New York, Los Angeles, Chicago, Houston, Detroit and Philadelphia.

The following discussion focuses on several white ethnic groups and attempts to describe some of the history of their migration to America, the areas where they now live, the common beliefs regarding health and illness, some kernels of information regarding family and social life, and problems that members from a given group may have in interacting with health care providers. The intention is not to create a vehicle for stereotyping but to whet the reader's appetite to search out more information about the people in their care, given the vast differences among Whites. There are countless cultural phenomena affecting health care.

■ German Americans

The following material, relating to both the German American and Polish American communities, was obtained from research conducted in southeastern Texas in May 1982 and updated over time. It is by no means indicative of the HEALTH and ILLNESS beliefs of the entire German American and Polish American communities. It is included here to demonstrate the type of data that can be gleaned using an "emic" (a description of behavior dependent on the person's categorization of the action) approach to collecting data. It cannot be generalized, but it allows the reader to grasp the diversity of beliefs that surround us (Lefcowitz, 1990, p. 6).

Since 1830 more than 7 million Germans have immigrated to the United States. There are presently 42.8 million Americans who claim German ancestry. Over 57.4% of the people 5 years and older speak German at home and 11.1% speak English less than very well. Thirty-nine percent of people of German ancestry reside in the Northeast and 39% reside in the South (U.S. Bureau of the Census, 2001, p. 46). The Germans represent a cross section of German society and have come from all social strata and walks of life. Some people have come to escape poverty, others have come for religious or political reasons, and still others have come to take advantage of the opportunity to open up the new lands. Many were recruited to come here, as were the Germans who settled in the German enclaves in Texas. The immigrants represented all religions, including primarily Lutherans, Catholics, and Jews. They represented the rich and the poor, the educated and the ignorant, and were of all ages. Present-day descendants are farmers, educators, and artists. The Germans brought to the United States the cultural diversity and folkways they observed in Germany. The festivals of Corpus Christi, Kinderfeste (children's feast), and Sangerfeste (singing festival) all originated in Germany (Conzen, 1980, pp. 405–425).

The Germans began to migrate to the United States in the 17th century and have contributed 15.2% of the total immigration population. They are the least visible ethnic group in the United States, and people often are surprised to discover that there is such a large Germanic influence in this country. In some places, the German communities maintain strong identification with their German heritage. For example, the city of Fredericksberg, Texas, maintains an ambience of German culture and identity. Some people born there who are fourth-generation and more continue to learn German as their first spoken language (Spector, 1983).

The German ethnic community is the second largest in the state of Texas and is exceeded only by the Mexican community. Germans have been immigrating to Texas since 1840 and continue to arrive. They are predominantly Catholic, Lutheran, and Methodist. Many of these people have maintained their German identity. The major German communities in Texas are Victoria, Cuero, Gonzales, New Braunfels, and Fredericksberg.

During the European freedom revolutions of 1830 and 1848, Texas was quite popular, especially in Germany, and was seen as a "wild and fabulous land." For tradition-bound German families, however, the abandonment of the homeland was difficult. They were enticed, however, by the hopes of economic and social improvement and political idealism. An additional reason for the mass migration was the overpopulation of Germany and the immigrants' desire to escape an imminent European catastrophe. By the 1840s, several thousand northern Germans had come to Texas, and another large migration occurred in 1890. This second cluster of people came because there was a severe crop failure in Russian-occupied Germany, and the Russian language had become a required subject in German schools. Other German migrations occurred from 1903 to 1905.

The Germans found pleasure in the small things of everyday life. They were tied together by the German language because it bound them to the past, entertaining them with games, riddles, folk songs and literature, and folk wisdom. The greatest amusement was singing and dancing. Religion for the Lutherans, Catholics, and Methodists was a part of everyday life. The year was measured by the church calendar; observance of church ritual paced the milestones of the life cycle. The Germans believed that each individual was a "part of the fabric of humanity," that "history was a continued process," and "everything had a purpose as mankind strove to something better" (Lich, 1982, pp. 33–72).

The Germans had a penchant for forming societies and clubs, the longest-lasting of which are the singing societies. The first was organized in 1850 and exists still today. The Germans brought with them their customs and traditions; their cures, curses, and recipes; and their tools and ways of building (Lich, 1982).

Health and Illness

Among the Germans, health is described as more than not being ill but as a state of well-being—physically and emotionally—the ability to do your duty, positive energy to do things, and the ability to do, think, and act the way you would like, to go and congregate, to enjoy life. Illness may be described as the absence of well-being: pain, malfunction of body organs, not being able to do what you want, a blessing from God to suffer, and a disorder of body, imbalance.

Causes of Illness

Most German Americans believe in the germ theory of infection and in stress-related theories. Other causes of illness are identified, however, such as drafts, environmental changes, and belief in the evil eye and punishment from God.

The methods of maintaining health include the requirement of dressing properly for the season, proper nutrition, and the wearing of shawls to protect oneself from drafts—also, the taking of cod-liver oil, exercise, and hard work. Methods for preventing illness include wearing an asafetida bag around the neck in the winter to prevent colds, scapulars, religious practices, sleeping with the windows open, and cleanliness.

Current Health Problems

There do not appear to be any unusual health problems particular to German Americans.

▓ Italian Americans

The Italian American community is made up of immigrants who came here from mainland Italy and from Sicily, Sardinia, and other Mediterranean islands that are part of Italy. The number of Americans claiming Italian ancestry is over 14.6 million. Over 77% of the people 5 years and older speak Italian at home and 39.6% speak English less than very well. Fifty-one percent of people of Italian ancestry reside in the Northeast (U.S. Bureau of the Census, 2001, p. 46).

Italian Americans indeed have a proud heritage in the United States, for America was "founded" by an Italian—Christopher Columbus; named for an Italian—Amerigo Vespucci; and explored by several Italian explorers, including Verrazano, Cabot, and Tonti (Bernardo, 1981, p. 26).

History of Migration

Between 1820 and 1990, over 5 million people from Italy immigrated to the United States (Lefcowitz, 1990, p. 6). The peak years were from 1901 to 1920, and only a small number of people continue to come today. Italians came to this country to escape poverty and to search for a better life in a country where they expected to reap rewards for their hard labor. The early years were not easy, but people chose to remain in this country and not return to Italy. Italians tended to live in neighborhood enclaves, and these neighborhoods, such as the North End in Boston and Little Italy in New York, still exist as Italian neighborhoods. Although the younger generation may have moved out, they still return home to maintain family, community, and ethnic ties (Nelli, 1980, pp. 545–560).

The family has served as the main tie keeping Italian Americans together because it provides its members with the strength to cope with the surrounding world and produces a sense of continuity in all situations. The family is the primary focus of the Italian's concern, and Italians take pride in the family and the home. Italians are resilient, yet fatalistic, and they take advantage of the present. Many upwardly mobile third- and fourth-generation Italian Americans often experience conflict between familial solidarity and society's emphasis on individualization and autonomy (Giordano & McGoldrick, 1996, p. 571). As mentioned, the home is a source of great pride, and it is a symbol of the family, not a status symbol per se. The church also is an important focus for the life of the Italian. Many of the festivals and observances continue to exist today, and in the summer, the North End of Boston is alive each weekend with the celebration of a different saint.

The father traditionally has been the head of the Italian household, and the mother is said to be the heart of the household.

Italian Americans have tended to attain low levels of education in the United States, but their incomes are comparable to or higher than those of other groups.

The Italian population falls into four generational groups: (1) the elderly, living in Italian enclaves; (2) a second generation, living both within the neighborhoods and in the suburbs; (3) a younger, well-educated group, living mainly in the suburbs; and (4) new immigrants (Ragucci, 1981, p. 216). More than 80% of Italian Americans marry people from a different ethnic group (Giordano & McGoldrick, 1996).

HEALTH and ILLNESS

Italians tend to present their symptoms to their fullest point and to expect immediate treatment for ailments. In terms of traditional beliefs, they may view the cause of illness to be one of the following: (1) winds and currents that bear diseases, (2) contagion or contamination, (3) heredity, (4) supernatural or human causes, and (5) psychosomatic interactions.

One such traditional Italian belief contends that moving air, in the form of drafts, causes irritation and then a cold that can lead to pneumonia. A belief an elderly person may express in terms of cancer surgery is that it is not a good idea to have surgery because surgery exposes the inner body to the air, and if the cancer is exposed to the air the person is going to die quicker. Just as drafts are considered to be a cause of illness, fresh air is considered to be vital for the maintenance of health. Homes and the workplace must be well ventilated to prevent illness from occurring.

One sees a belief in contamination manifested in the reluctance of people to share food and objects with people who are considered unclean, and often in not entering the homes of those who are ill. Traditional Italian women have a strong sense of modesty and shame, resulting in an avoidance of discussions relating to sex and menstruation.

Blood is regarded by some, especially the elderly, to be a "plastic entity" that responds to fluids and food and is responsible for many variable conditions. Various adjectives, such as *high* and *low* and *good* and *bad*, are used to describe blood. Some of the "old superstitions" include the following beliefs:

1. Congenital abnormalities can be attributed to the unsatisfied desire for food during pregnancy.
2. If a pregnant woman is not given food that she smells, the fetus will move inside, and a miscarriage will result.
3. If a pregnant woman bends, turns, or moves in a certain way, the fetus may not develop normally.
4. A woman must not reach during pregnancy because reaching can harm the fetus.

Italians may also attribute the cause of illness to the evil eye (*malocchio*) or to curses (*castiga*). The difference between these two causes is that less serious illnesses, such as headaches, may be caused by *malocchio*, whereas more severe illness, which often can be fatal, may be attributed to more powerful *castiga*. Curses are sent either by God or by evil people. An example of a curse is the punishment from God for sins and bad behavior (Ragucci, 1981, p. 216).

Italians recognize that illness can be caused by the suppression of emotions, as well as stress from fear, grief, and anxiety. If one is unable to find an emotional outlet, one well may "burst." It is not considered healthy to bottle up emotions (Ragucci, 1981, p. 232).

Often, the care of the ill is managed in the home, with all members of the family sharing in the responsibilities. The use of home remedies ostensibly is decreasing, although several students have reported the continued use of rituals for the removal of the evil eye and the practice of leeching. One practice described for the removal of the evil eye was to take an egg and olive oil and to drip them into a pan of water, make the sign of the cross, and recite prayers. If the oil spreads over the water, the cause of the problem is the evil eye, and the illness should get better. Mineral waters are also used, and tonics are used to cleanse the blood. There is a strong religious influence among Italians, who believe that faith in God and the saints will see them through the illness. One woman whom I worked with had breast cancer. She had had surgery several years before and did not have a recurrence. She attributed her recovery to the fact that she attended mass every morning and that she had total faith in Saint Peregrine, whose medal she wore pinned to her bra by the site of the mastectomy. Italian people tend to take a fatalistic stance regarding terminal illness and death, believing that it is God's will. Death often is not discussed between the dying person and the family members. I recall when caring for an elderly Italian man at home that it was not possible to have the man and his wife discuss his impending death. Although both knew that he was dying and would talk with the nurse, to each other he "was going to recover," and everything possible was done to that end.

Italian families observe numerous religious traditions surrounding death, and funeral masses and anniversary masses are observed. It is the custom for the widow to wear black for some time after her husband's death (occasionally for the remainder of her life), although this is not as common with the younger generations.

Health-Related Problems

Two genetic diseases commonly seen among Italians are (1) favism, a severe hemolytic anemia caused by deficiency of the X-linked enzyme glucose-6-phosphate dehydrogenase and triggered by the eating of fava beans, and (2) the thalassemia syndromes, also hemolytic anemias that include Cooley's anemia (or beta-thalassemia) and alpha-thalassemia (Ragucci, 1981, p. 222).

Language problems frequently occur when elderly or new Italian immigrants are seeking care. Often, due to modesty, people are reluctant to answer the questions asked through interpreters, and gathering of pertinent data is very difficult.

Problems related to time also occur. Physicians tend to diagnose emotional problems more often for Italian patients than for other ethnic groups because of the Italian pattern of reporting more symptoms and reporting them more dramatically (Giordano & McGoldrick, 1996, p. 576).

In general, Italian Americans are motivated to seek explanations with respect to their health status and the care they are to receive. If instructions and explanations are well given, Italians tend to cooperate with health care providers. It is often necessary to provide directions in the greatest detail and then to provide written instructions to ensure compliance with necessary regimens.

Polish Americans

The first people immigrating to this country from Poland came with Germans in 1608 to Jamestown, Virginia, to help develop the timber industry. Since that time, Poland, too, has given America one of its largest ethnic groups, with over 9 million people claiming Polish ancestry. The peak year for Polish immigration was 1921, and well over 578,875 people immigrated here. Many of the people arriving before 1890 came for economic reasons. Those coming here since that time have come for both economic and political reasons and for religious freedom. Polish heroes include Casimir Pulaski and Thaddeus Kosciuszko, who were heroes in the American Revolution. The major influx of Poles to the United States began in 1870 and ended in 1913. The people who arrived were mainly peasants seeking food and release from the political oppression of three foreign governments in Poland. The immigrants who came both before and after this mass migration were better educated and not as poor. In the United States, Polish immigrants lived in poor conditions either because they had no choice or because that was the way they were able to meet their own priorities. They were seen by other Americans to live as animals and were often mocked and called stupid. Quite often, the Polish people spoke and understood several European languages but had difficulty learning English and were therefore scorned. Polish people shared the problem as a community and banded together in tight enclaves called "Polonia." They attempted to be as self-sufficient as possible. They worked at preserving their native culture, and voluntary Polish ghettos grew up in close proximity to the parish church (Green, 1980, pp. 787–803). Over 85.5% of those 5 years and older speak Polish at home and 50.3% speak English less than very well. Thirty-seven percent of people of Polish ancestry reside in the Northeast, as well as 37% in the Midwest (U.S. Bureau of the Census, 2001, p. 46).

An example of the Polish experience in the United States is that of the Polish immigrants in Texas. The first Poles came to Texas in the second half of the 19th century, and most of them settled in Victoria, San Antonio, Houston, and Bandera. The first Polish colonies in America were located in Texas, the oldest being Panna Maria (Virgin Mary) in Karnes County, 50 miles southeast of San Antonio. Unlike other Poles who wanted to return to Poland, the colonists who arrived in Texas after 1850 came to settle permanently and had no intention of returning to their homeland. Although these people came to Texas for economic, political, and religious reasons, severe poverty was their major reason for leaving Poland.

The first collective Polish immigration to America was in 1854, when 100 families came to Texas. They landed in Galveston, where a few in the party remained. The rest traveled in a procession northwestward, taking with them a few belongings, such as featherbeds, crude farm implements, and a cross from their parish church. Their dream was to live in the fertile lands of Texas and raise crops, speak their own language, educate their children, and worship God as they pleased. This dream did not materialize, and members of the band grew discouraged. Some of the immigrants remained in Victoria and others went to San Antonio.

The people who went to San Antonio continued to travel; on Christmas Eve, 1854, they stopped at the junction of the San Antonio and Cibolo Rivers; There, under a live oak tree, they celebrated mass and founded Panna Maria. In 1855, 1856, and 1857, others followed this small group in moving to this part of Texas.

These settlers were exposed to many dangers from nature, such as heat, drought, snakes, and insects. The Polish settlers were not accepted by the other settlers in the area because their language, customs, and culture were different, but the immigrants survived, and many moved to settle other areas near Panna Maria. Today, the people of Panna Maria continue to live simple lives close to nature and God and speak mainly Polish.

Much of the history of the Polish people in Texas is written around the founding and the location of the various church parishes. For example, in 1873 the Parish of the Nativity of the Blessed Virgin Mary was begun in Cestohowa. Within this church above the main altar is a large picture of the Virgin Mary of Czestochowa. This picture was taken to the church from Panna Maria. It is a copy of the famous Black Madonna of Czestochowa, Poland, a city 65 miles east of where the immigrants to Texas originated. The Black Madonna is a beloved, miraculous image and a source of faith to the Polish people. The Shrine of Our Lady in Czestochowa, Poland, is one of the largest shrines in the world. Since the 14th century, that picture had been the object of veneration and devotion of Polish Catholics. It is claimed to have been painted by Saint Luke the Evangelist. Its origin is traced to the 5th or 6th century and is the oldest picture of the Virgin in the world. The scars on the face date from 1430, when bandits struck it with a sword. The history, traditions, and miracles of Czestochowa are the heritage of the Polish people (Dworaczyk, 1979). One woman I interviewed said she had been ill with a fatal disease. The entire time that she lay close to death she prayed to the Virgin. When she finally did recover, she made a pilgrimage back to her homeland in Poland and visited the shrine to give thanks to the Virgin. The woman was positive that this was the source of her recovery.

HEALTH and ILLNESS

The definitions of HEALTH among the Polish people I interviewed included "feeling okay—as a whole—body, spirit, everything a person cannot separate;" happy, until war, do not need doctor, do not need medicine; "active, able to work, feel good, do what I want to do;" and "good spirit, good to everybody, never cross." The definitions of ILLNESS may include "something wrong with body, mind, or spirit;" "one wrong affects them all;" "not capable of working, see the doctor often;" "not right, something ailing you;" "not active"; "feeling bad"; and "opposite of health, not doing what I want to do." The methods for maintaining HEALTH include maintaining a happy home, being kind and loving, eating healthy food, remaining pure, walking, exercising, wearing proper clothing (sweaters), eating a well-balanced diet, trying not to worry, having faith in God, being active, dressing warmly, going to bed early, and working hard. The methods for preventing ILLNESS include cleanliness, the wearing of scapulars, avoiding drafts, following the proper diet, not gossiping, keeping away from people with colds, and wearing medals because "God is with you all the time to protect you and take care of you." Other ideas about ILLNESS include the beliefs that ILLNESSES are caused by poor diets and that the evil eye may well exist as a causative factor. This belief was attributed to the older generations and is not regarded as prevalent among younger Polish Americans.

Health Care Problems

The Polish community has not tended to have any major problems with health care deliverers. Language may be a barrier if members of the older generation do not speak English, and the taking of health histories is complicated when the providers cannot communicate directly with the informant. Again, problems may develop when there is difficulty finding someone who is conversant in Polish whom the informant can trust to reveal personal matters to and who can translate medical terms accurately.

In Poland, there is a shortage of medical supplies, so the people tend to use faith healers and believe in miracle workers. On the main street of Warsaw all sorts of folk medicine and miracle-worker paraphernalia are on sale: divining rods, cotton sacks filled with herbs to be worn over an ailing heart or liver, coils of copper wire to be placed under food to rid it of poisons, and pendulums (*Letter from Poland,* 1983).

■ Health Status of White Population

There are countless health status indicators wherein the White cohort of the population differs from the total population, each of the racial groups, and Hispanics as the populations were designated by Census 2000. In each of the preceding four chapters, there has been a table comparing the relevant group and all races. In this chapter it is appropriate to compare the White populations to all races and to specific populations. In spite of the fact that only 13 health indicators are listed as examples in the tables, the health differences and disparities in the overall populations are readily apparent.

Table 10–1 lists the 10 leading causes of death for Whites and compares them with the causes of death for the general population in 2004.

In this chapter, as in this entire book, I have attempted to open the door to the enormous diversity in health and illness beliefs that exists in White (European American) communities specifically and in the entire American population in general. I have only opened the door and invited you to peek inside. There is a richness of knowledge to be gained. It is for you to acquire it as you care for all

Table 10-1 Comparison of the 10 Leading Causes of Death for White Americans and for All Persons: 2004

White Americans	All Persons
1. Diseases of heart	Diseases of heart
2. Malignant neoplasms	Malignant neoplasms
3. Cerebrovascular diseases	Cerebrovascular diseases
4. Chronic lower respiratory diseases	Chronic lower respiratory diseases
5. Unintentional injuries	Unintentional injuries
6. Alzheimer's disease	Diabetes mellitus
7. Diabetes mellitus	Alzheimer's disease
8. Influenza and pneumonia	Influenza and pneumonia
9. Nephritis, nephrotic syndrome, and nephrosis	Nephritis, nephrotic syndrome, and nephrosis
10. Suicide	Septicemia

Source: National Center for Health Statistics. (2007). *Health, United States, 2007 with chartbook on trends in the health of Americans* (p. 187). Hyattsville, MD: Author.

patients. Ask them what they believe about health/HEALTH and illness/ILLNESS and what their traditional beliefs, practices, and remedies are. The students whom I am working with find this to be a very enlightening experience.

Explore 🌐 MediaLink

Go to the Companion Website at www.prenhall.com/spector for chapter-related review questions, case studies, and activities. Contents of the CulturalCare Guide and CulturalCare Museum can also be found on the Companion Website. Click on Chapter 12 to select the activities for this chapter.

▓ Internet Sources

Brittingham, A., and de la Cruz, G. P. Ancestry: 2000 Census Brief (2004). Washington: DC: United States Census Bureau, pp. 1–2. Retrieved from https://ask.census.gov/cgi-bin/askcensus.cfg. February 23, 2008.

Grieco, E. M. (2001). The White Population: 2000. Washington, DC: U.S. Census Bureau. P. 7 Retrieved from http://www.census.gov/population/www/cen2000/briefs.html, February 23, 2008.

Larsen, L. J. (2004). *The Foreign-Born Population in the United States: 2003.* Washington, DC: U.S. Census Bureau. p.1 Retrieved from http://www.census.gov/prod/2004pubs/p20–551.pdf, May 23, 2008.

U.S. Census Bureau, Census 2000 Special Tabulations. Profile of Selected Demographic and Social Characteristics: 2000 United States, Germany, Italy, and Poland. Retrieved from http://factfinder.census.gov, http://www.census.gov/population/cen2000/stp-159/STP-159-Europe.pdf, http://www.census.gov/population/cen2000/stp-159/STP-159-Germany.pdf, http://www.census.gov/ population/cen2000/stp-159/STP-159Italy.pdf, http://www.census.gov/population/cen2000/stp-159/STP-159-Poland.pdf, February 23, 2008.

References

Bernardo, S. (1981). *The ethnic almanac.* New York: Doubleday.

Conzen, K. N. (1980). Germans. In S. Thernstrom (Ed.), *Harvard encyclopedia of American ethnic groups* (pp. 405–425). Cambridge, MA: Harvard University Press.

Dworaczyk, E. J. (1979). *The first Polish colonies of America in Texas.* San Antonio, TX: Naylor.

Folwarski, J., & Marganoff, P. P. (1996). Polish families. In M. McGoldrick, J. Giordano, & J. K. Pearce (Eds.), *Ethnicity and family therapy* (2nd ed.). New York: Guilford.

Giordano, J., & McGoldrick, M. (1996). Italian families. In M. McGoldrick, J. Giordano, & J. K. Pearce (Eds.), *Ethnicity and family therapy* (2nd ed.). New York: Guilford.

Green, V. (1980). Poles. In S. Thernstrom (Ed.), *Harvard encyclopedia of American ethnic groups.* Cambridge, MA: Harvard University Press.

Lefcowitz, E. (1990). *The United States immigration history timeline.* New York: Terra Firma Press.

Letter from Poland—of faith healers and miracle workers. (1983, August 21). *Boston Globe,* p.

Lich, G. E. (1982). *The German Texan.* San Antonio: University of Texas Institute of Texan Cultures.

Lollock, L. (2000). *The foreign-born population in the United States.* Washington, DC: U.S. Bureau of the Census.

Meyer, J. (2001). *Age: 2000.* Washington, DC: U.S. Census Bureau.

National Center for Health Statistics, et al. (2001). *Health, United States, 2001 urban and rural health chartbook.* Hyattsville, MD: Author.

National Center for Health Statistics. (2006). *Health, United States, 2006 with chartbook on trends in the health of Americans.* Hyattsville, MD: Author.

Nelli, H. S. (1980). Italians. In S. Thernstrom (Ed.), *Harvard encyclopedia of American ethnic groups.* Cambridge, MA: Harvard University Press.

Ragucci, A. T. (1981). Italian Americans. In A. Harwood (Ed.), *Ethnicity and medical care.* Cambridge, MA: Harvard University Press.

Spector, R. E. (1983). *A description of the impact of Medicare on health-illness beliefs and practices of White ethnic senior citizens in Central Texas.* PhD. diss. University Texas at Austin School of Nursing, Ann Arbor, MI: University Microfilms International.

Spector, R. (1992). Culture, ethnicity, and nursing. In P. Potter & A. Perry (Eds.), *Fundamentals of nursing* (3rd ed.). St Louis: Mosby.

U.S. Bureau of the Census. (2001). *Statistical abstract of the United States: 2001.* Washington, DC: Author.

Winawer, H., & Wetzel, N. A. (1996). German families. In M. McGoldrick, J. Giordano, & J. K. Pearce (Eds.), *Ethnicity and family therapy* (2nd ed.). New York: Guilford.

Epilogue

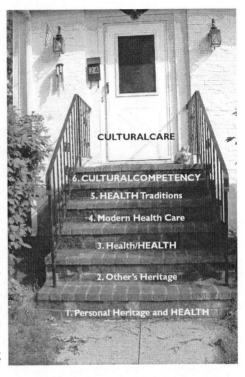

CULTURALCARE

6. CULTURALCOMPETENCY

5. HEALTH Traditions

4. Modern Health Care

3. Health/HEALTH

2. Other's Heritage

1. Personal Heritage and HEALTH

Why must health care deliverers—nurses, physicians, public health and social workers, and other health care professionals—study culture, ethnicity, religion, and become CULTURALLY COMPETENT? Why must they know the difference between *hot* and *cold* and *yin* and *yang*? Why must they be concerned with the patient's failure to practice what professionals believe to be good preventive medicine or with the patient's failure to follow a given treatment regimen or with the patient's failure to seek medical care during the initial phase of an illness? Is there a difference between curing and HEALING?

There is little disagreement that health care services in this country are unevenly distributed and that the poor and the emerging majority get the short end of the stick in terms of the care they receive (or do not receive). The apparent health disparities are a reality, as are the demographic and social disparities in areas of housing, employment, education, and opportunity. Just as there is the need to understand the people who constitute our multicultural society, there is also the need to understand new immigrants as more and more people flock to this country. However, it is often maintained that, when health care is provided, people fail to use it or use it inappropriately. Why is this seeming paradox so?

The major focus of this book has been on the provider's and the patient's differing perceptions of health/HEALTH and illness/ILLNESS. These differences may account for the health care provider's misconception that services are used inappropriately and that people do not care about their health/HEALTH. What to the casual observer appears to be "misuse" may represent our failure to understand and to meet the needs and expectations of the patient. This possibility may well be difficult for health care providers to face, but careful analysis of the available information seems to indicate that this may—at least in part—be the case. How, then, can we who are health care providers change our method of operations and provide both safe and effective care for the emerging majority and, at the same time, for the population at large? The answer to this question is not an easy one, and some researchers think we are not succeeding. A number of measures can and must be taken to ameliorate the current situation. CULTUR-ALCARE and the educational preparation leading to this is a **process,** one that becomes a way of life and must be recognized as such. This is a philosophical issue. The changing of one's personal and professional philosophies, ideas, and stereotypes does *not* occur overnight, and the process, quite often, is neither direct nor easy. It is a multistep process, in which one must

- Explore one's own cultural identity and heritage and confront biases and stereotypes.
- Develop an awareness and understanding of the complexities of the modern health care delivery system—its philosophy and problems, biases, and stereotypes.
- Develop a keen awareness of the socialization process that brings the provider into this complex system.
- Develop the ability to "hear" things that transcend language and foster an understanding of the patient and his or her cultural heritage and the resilience found within the culture that supports family and community structures.

I should like to reiterate that this book was written with the hope that, by sharing the material I have learned and taught for over 35 years, some small changes will be made in the thinking of all health care providers who read it. There is nothing new in these pages. Perhaps it is simply a recombination of material with which the reader is familiar, but I hope it serves its purpose: the sharing of beliefs and attitudes and the stimulation of lots of consciousness raising concerning issues of vital concern to health care providers who must confront the needs of patients with diverse cultural backgrounds.

Appendix A

Selected Key Terms Related to Cultural Diversity in HEALTH and ILLNESS

The following terms have been defined to help you in the development of CULTURALCOMPETENCY. They are the "bricks" that comprise the steps that must be climbed. They are the language of CULTURALCARE.

Aberglaubish or *aberglobin*—The traditional German term for the "evil eye."

Access—Gaining entry into a system—the term used in this text refers to access into the modern health care system. *Access* also means entry into a profession, education, employment, housing, and so forth.

Acculturation—The process of adapting to another culture. To acquire the majority group's culture.

Acupuncture—The traditional Chinese medical way of restoring the balance of *yin* and *yang* that is based on the therapeutic value of cold. Cold is used in a disease where there is an excess of *yang*.

Alcoholismo—Alcoholism.

Alien—Every person applying for entry to the United States. Anyone who is not a U.S. citizen.

Allopathic—Health beliefs and practices that are derived from current scientific models and involve the use of technology and other modalities of present-day health care, such as immunization, proper nutrition, and resuscitation.

Allopathy—The treatment of a disease by using remedies that cause the opposite effects of the disease.

Alternative health system—A system of health care a person may use that is not predicated within his or her traditional culture but is not allopathic.

Amulet—An object with magical powers, such as a charm, worn on a string or chain around the neck, wrist, or waist to protect the wearer from both physical and psychic illness, harm, and misfortune.

Anamnesis—The traditional Chinese medical way of diagnosing a health problem by asking questions.

Apparel—Traditional clothing worn by people for cultural or religious beliefs on a daily basis, such as head coverings.

Aromatherapy—Ancient science that uses essential plant oils to produce strong physical and emotional effects in the body.

Assimilation—To become absorbed into another culture and to adopt its characteristics. To develop a new cultural identity.

Ataque de nervios—An attack of nerves or a nervous breakdown.

Average charge—Average amount of monetary charge in hospital bills for discharged patients.

Average length of stay—The typical number of days a patient stays in the hospital for a particular condition.

Ayurvedic—Four-thousand-year-old method of healing originating in India, the chief aim of which is longevity and quality of life. The most ancient existing medical system that uses diet, natural therapies, and herbs.

Bankes—Small, bell-shaped glass that is used to create a vacuum, placed on a person's chest, to loosen chest secretions.

Biofeedback—The use of an electronic machine to measure skin temperatures. The patient controls responses that are usually involuntary.

Biological variations—Biological differences that exist among races and ethnic groups in body structure, skin color, biochemical differences, susceptibility to disease, and nutritional differences.

Borders—Legal, geographic separations between nations.

Botanica—Traditional Hispanic pharmacy where amulets, herbal remedies, books, candles, and statues of saints may be purchased.

Bruja—A witch.

Caida de la mollera (**fallen fontanel**)—Traditional Hispanic belief that the fontanel falls if the baby's head is touched.

Calendar—Dates of religious holidays. Many of these dates of observance can change from year to year on the Julian calendar.

Care—Factors that assist, enable, support, or facilitate a person's needs to maintain, improve, or ease a health problem.

Celos—Jealousy.

Charm—Objects that combine the functions of both amulets and talismans but consist only of written words or symbols.

Chinese doctor—Physician educated in China who uses traditional herbs and other therapeutic modalities in the delivery of health care.

Chiropractic—A form of health care that believes in the use of "energy" to treat diseases.

Complementary medicine—Treatment modalities used to complement allopathic regimens.

Conjure—To effect magic.

Coraje—Rage.

Costs—The monetary price of an item or the consequences of ignoring social factors.

CULTURALCARE—A concept that describes holistic HEALTH care that is culturally sensitive, culturally appropriate, and culturally competent. CULTURALCARE is critical to meeting the complex nursing care needs of a person, family, and community. It is the provision of health care across cultural boundaries and takes into account the context in which the patient lives as well as the situations in which the patient's health problems arise.

Culturally appropriate—Implies that the health care provider applies the underlying background knowledge that must be possessed to provide a given patient with the best possible HEALTH care.

CULTURALLY COMPETENT—Implies that within the delivered care the health care provider understands and attends to the total context of the patient's situation. CULTURALCOMPETENCE is a complex combination of knowledge, attitudes, and skills.

Culturally sensitive—Implies that the health care providers possess some basic knowledge of and constructive attitudes toward the HEALTH traditions observed among the diverse cultural groups found in the setting in which they are practicing.

Culture—Nonphysical traits, such as values, beliefs, attitudes, and customs, that are shared by a group of people and passed from one generation to the next. A metacommunication system.

Culture shock—Disorder that occurs in response to transition from one cultural setting to another. Former behavior patterns are ineffective in such a setting, and basic cues for social behavior are absent.

Curandero—Traditional Hispanic holistic healer.

Curing˙—Two-dimensional phenomenon that results in ridding the body or mind (or both) of a given disease.

Decoction—A simmered tea made from the bark, root, seed, or berry of a plant.

Demographic disparity—A variation below the percentages of the profile of the total population with a specific entity, such as poverty, or professional, such as nursing. Comparison with the demographic profile of the total population.

Demographic parity—An equal distribution of a given entity, such as registered nurses, and the demographic profile of the total population.

Demographics—The population profile of the nation, state, county, or local city or town.

Demography—The statistical study of populations, including statistical counts of people of various ages, sexes, and population densities for specific locations.

Determinism—Believing that life is under a person's control.

Diagnosis—The identifying of the nature or cause of something, especially a problem.

Disadvantaged background—Both educational and economic factors that act as barriers to an individual's participation in a health professions program.

Discrimination—Denying people equal opportunity by acting on a prejudice.

Divination—Traditional American Indian practice of calling on spirits or other forces to determine a diagnosis of a health problem.

Documentation—The papers necessary to prove one's citizenship or immigration status.

Duklij—A turquoise or green malachite amulet that may be used among American Indians to ward off evil spirits.

Dybbuk—Wandering, disembodied soul that enters another person's body and holds fast.

Emerging majority—People of color—Blacks; Asians/Pacific Islanders; American Indians, Eskimos, or Aleuts; and Hispanics—who are expected to constitute a majority of the American population by the year 2020.

Emic—Person's way of describing an action or event, an inside view.

Empacho—Traditional Hispanic belief that a ball of food is stuck in the stomach.

Envidia—Traditional Hispanic belief that the envy of others can be the cause of illness and bad luck.

Environmental control—Ability of a person from a given cultural group to actively control nature and to direct factors in the environment.

Epidemiology—The study of the distribution of disease.

Epilepsia—Epilepsy.

Ethnicity—Cultural group's sense of identification associated with the group's common social and cultural heritage.

Ethnocentrism—Tendency of members of one cultural group to view the members of other cultural groups in terms of the standards of behavior, attitudes, and values of their own group. The belief that one's own cultural, ethnic, professional, or social group is superior to that of others.

Ethnomedicine—Health beliefs and practices of indigenous cultural development. Not practiced in many of the tenets of modern medicine.

Etic—The interpretation of an event by someone who is not experiencing that event. An outside view.

Evil eye—Belief that someone can project harm by gazing or staring at another's property or person.

Excessism—Desiring to live with numerous possessions and material goods.

Exorcism—Ceremonious expulsion of an evil spirit from a person.

Faith—Strong beliefs in a religious or other spiritual philosophy.

Fatalism—Believing that life is not under a person's control.

Fatigue—Asthmalike symptoms.

Folklore—Body of preserved traditions, usually oral, consisting of beliefs, stories, and associated information of people.

Fundamentalism—Strict belief in the traditions of a heritage.

Geophagy—Eating of nonfood substances, such as starch.

Glossoscopy—Traditional Chinese medical way of diagnosing a health problem by examining the tongue.

Green card—Documentation that a person is a legally admitted immigrant and has permanent resident status in the United States.

Gris-gris—Symbols of voodoo. They may take numerous forms and be used either to protect a person or to harm that person.

Halal—A designation for meat from animals that has been slaughtered in the ritual way by Islamic law so that it is suitable to be eaten by traditional Islamic people and follows Islamic dietary laws.

Haragei—Japanese art of practice of using nonverbal communication.

HEALING*—Holistic, or three-dimensional, phenomenon that results in the restoration of balance, or harmony, to the body, mind, and spirit, or between the person and the environment.

HEALTH*—The balance of the person, both within one's being—physical, mental, and spiritual—and in the outside world—natural, communal, and metaphysical.

Herbrias—A person who sells herbs.

Heritage—The family culture, ethnicity, and/or religion that one is born into.

Heritage consistency—Observance of the beliefs and practices of one's traditional cultural belief system.

Heritage inconsistency—Observance of the beliefs and practices of one's acculturated belief system.

Hex—Evil spell, misfortune, or bad luck that one person can impose on another.

Histeria—Hysteria.

Homeopathic—Health beliefs and practices derived from traditional cultural knowledge to maintain health, prevent changes in health status, and restore health.

Homeopathic medicine—In the practice of homeopathic medicine, the person, not the disease, is treated.

Homeopathy—System of medicine based on the belief that a disease can be cured by minute doses of a substance, which, if given to a healthy person in large doses, would produce the same symptoms that the person being treated is experiencing.

Hoodoo—A form of conjuring and a term that refers to the magical practices of voodoo outside New Orleans.

Hydrotherapy—The use of water in the maintenance of health and treatment of disease.

Hypnotherapy—The use of hypnosis to stimulate emotions and control involuntary responses, such as blood pressure.

Iatrogenic—The unexpected symptom or illness that can result from the treatment of another illness.

ILLNESS*—State of imbalance among the body, mind, and spirit. A sense of disharmony both within the person and with the environment.

Immigrant—Alien entering the United States for permanent (or temporary) residence.

Indigenous—People native to an area.

Kineahora—Word spoken by traditional Jewish people to prevent the "evil eye."

Kosher—A designation for food that has been prepared so that it is suitable to be eaten by traditional Jewish people and follows Jewish dietary laws.

Kusiut—A reference term for an American Indian medicine man. A "learned one."

Lay midwife—A person who practices lay midwifery.

Lay midwifery—Assisting childbirth for compensation.

Legal Permanent Resident (LPR)—Green card recipient. A person who has been granted lawful permanent residence in the United States.

Limpia—Traditional Hispanic practice of cleansing a person.

Locura—Craziness.

Macrobiotics—Diet and lifestyle from the Far East adapted for the United States by Michio Kushif. The principles of this vegetarian diet consist of balancing *yin* and *yang* energies of food.

Magico-religious folk medicine—Use of charms, holy words, and holy actions to prevent and cure illness.

Mal ojo (**bad eye**)—Traditional Hispanic belief that excessive admiration by one person can bring harm to another person.

Massage therapy—Use of manipulative techniques to relieve pain and return energy to the body.

Materialism—Taking great pleasure from having more than is necessary.

Medically underserved community—Urban or rural population group that lacks adequate health care services.

Melting pot—The social blending of cultures.

Meridians—Specific points of the body into which needles are inserted in the traditional Chinese medical practice of acupuncture.

Mesmerism—Healing by touch.

Metacommunication system—Large system of communication that includes both verbal language and nonverbal signs and symbols.

Milagros—Small figures of body parts or other objects that are offered to Saints for thanksgiving.

Minimalism—Knowing how to live with few possessions and material goods.

Miracle—Supernatural, unexplained event.

Modern—Present-day health and illness beliefs and practices of the providers within the American, or Western, health care delivery system.

Modernism—Adherence to modern ways and a belief that other values no longer exist.

Motion in the hand—An example of a traditional American Indian practice of moving the diagnostician's hands in a ritual of divination.

Moxibustion—Traditional Chinese medical way of restoring the balance of *yin* and *yang* that is based on the therapeutic value of heat. Heat is used in a disease where there is an excess of *yin*.

Multicultural nursing—Pluralistic approach to understanding relationships between two or more cultures to create a nursing practice framework for broadening nurses' understanding of health-related beliefs, practices, and issues that are part of the experiences of people from diverse cultural backgrounds.

Mysticism—Aspect of spiritual healing and beliefs.

Natural folk medicine—Use of the natural environment and use of herbs, plants, minerals, and animal substances to prevent and treat illness.

Nonimmigrant—People who are allowed to enter the country temporarily under certain conditions, such as crewmen, students, and temporary workers.

Occult folk medicine—The use of charms, holy words, and holy actions to prevent and cure illness.

Orisha—Yoruba god or goddess.

Osphretics—Traditional Chinese medical way of diagnosing a health problem by listening and smelling.

Osteopathic medicine—School of medical practice that directs recuperative power of nature that is within the body to cure a disease.

Overheating therapy (hyperthermia)—Used since the time of the ancient Greeks. The natural immune system is stimulated with heat to kill pathogens.

Partera—A Mexican American or Mexican lay midwife.

Pasmo—Traditional Hispanic disease of paralysis, face or limbs.

Pluralistic society—A society comprising people of numerous ethnocultural backgrounds.

Poultice—A hot, soft, moist mass of herbs, flour, mustard, and other substances spread on muslin and placed on a sore body part.

Powwow—A form of traditional HEALING practiced by German Americans.

Prejudice—Negative beliefs or preferences that are generalized about a group and that leads to "prejudgment."

Promesa—A deep and serious promise.

Racism—The belief that members of one race are superior to those of other races.

Rational folk medicine—Use of the natural environment and use of herbs, plants, minerals, and animal substances to prevent and treat illness.

Raza-Latina—A popular term used as a reference group name for people of Latin American descent.

Reflexology—Natural science that manipulates the reflex points in the hands and feet that correspond to every organ in the body in order to clear the energy pathways and the flow of energy through the body.

Religion—Belief in a divine or superhuman power or powers to be obeyed and worshipped as the creator(s) and ruler(s) of the universe.

Remedies—Natural folk medicines that use the natural environment—herbs, plants, minerals, and animal substances to treat illnesses. Natural remedies have come to the United States from every corner of the world—the East and the West. They may be purchased in pharmacies, markets, and natural food stores.

Resident alien—A lawfully admitted alien.

Resiliency—The state of being strong and able to resist the consequences of an adverse event or emotional or physical danger.

Restoration—Process used by a person to return health.

Risk adjustment—Complex sets of data are put into terms whereby they are compared apples to apples.

Sacred objects—Objects, such as amulets and *milagros*, that have a spiritual purpose.

Sacred places—Places where people take petitions for favors or offer prayers of thanksgiving for the granting of a request.

Sacred practices—Religious practices, such as dietary taboos or lighting of candles, that a person is commanded to follow.

Santeria—A syncretic religion comprising both African and Catholic beliefs.

Santero(a)—Traditional priest and healer in the religion of *Santeria*.

Secular—Beliefs and practices that are not under the auspices of a religious body.

Self-denialism—Taking great pleasure from having less than is necessary.

Senoria—A woman who is knowledgeable about the causes and treatment of illness.

Sexism—Belief that members of one sex are superior to those of the other sex.

Shrine—A place—natural, secular, and/or affiliated with a religious tradition—where people make spiritual journeys or pilgrimages for the purposes of giving thanks or petitioning for favors. They are related to magico-religious folk medicine, and the use of charms, holy words, and holy actions, such as prayer, may be observed.

Singer—A type of traditional American Indian healer who is able to practice singing as a form of treating a health problem.

Skilly—An agent that is believed to cause disease by traditional Cherokee people.

Social organization—Patterns of cultural behavior related to life events, such as birth, death, childrearing, and health and illness, that are followed within a given social group.

Socialization—Process of being raised within a culture and acquiring the characteristics of the group.

Soul loss—Belief that a person's soul can leave the body, wander around, and then return.

Space—Area surrounding a person's body and the objects within that area.

Spell—A magical word or formula or a condition of evil or bad luck.

Sphygmopalpation—Traditional Chinese medical way of diagnosing a health problem by feeling pulses.

Spirit—The noncorporeal and nonmental dimension of a person that is the source of meaning and unity. The source of the experience of spirituality and every religion.

Spirit possession—Belief that a spirit can enter people, possess them, and control what they say and do.

Spiritual—Ideas, attitudes, concepts, beliefs, and behaviors that are the result of a person's experience of the spirit.

Spirituality—The experience of meaning and unity.

Stargazing—Example of a traditional American Indian practice of praying the star prayer to the star spirit as a method of divination.

Stereotype—Notion that all people from a given group are the same.

Superstition—Belief that performing an action, wearing a charm or an amulet, or eating something will have an influence on life events. These beliefs are upheld by magic and faith.

Susto (**soul loss**)—Traditional Hispanic belief that the soul is able to leave a person's body.

Szatan—The traditional Polish term for the "evil eye."

Taboo—A culture-bound ban that excludes certain behaviors from common use.

Talisman—Consecrated religious object that confers power of various kinds and protects people who wear, carry, or own them from harm and evil.

Tao—Way, path, or discourse. On the spiritual level, the way to ultimate reality.

Time—Duration, interval of time. Instances, points in time.

Tirisia—Anxiety.

Title VI—Under the provisions of Title VI of the Civil Rights Act of 1964, people with Limited English Proficiency (LEP) who are cared for in such health care settings as extended care facilities, public assistance programs, nursing homes, and hospitals and are eligible for Medicaid, other health care, or human services cannot be denied assistance because of their race, color, or national origin.

Traditional—Ancient, ethnocultural-religious beliefs and practices that have been handed down through the generations.

Traditional epidemiology—Belief in agents other than those of a scientific nature, causing disease. These could be such agents as "envy," "jealousy," and "hate."

Traditionalism—Belief in the traditional HEALTH, ILLNESS, and HEALING methods of a given cultural cohort.

Tui Na—A complex Chinese system of massage, "pushing and pulling," using meridian stimulation used to treat orthopedic and neurological problems.

Undocumented alien—Person of foreign origin who has entered the country unlawfully by bypassing inspection or who has overstayed the original terms of admission.

Universalism—Open beliefs in many domains that may not be part of a given personal heritage.

Unlocking—Steps taken to help break down and understand the definitions of the terms *health*/HEALTH and *illness*/ILLNESS in a living context. It consists of persistent questioning: What is health? No matter what the response, the question "What does that mean?" is asked. Initially, this causes much confusion, but as each term is analyzed the process makes sense.

Voodoo—A religion that is a combination of Christianity and African Yoruba religious beliefs.

Vulnerability—The state of being weak or prone to an adverse event or emotional or physical danger.

Witched—Example of a traditional American Indian belief that a person is harmed by witches.

Xenophobia—Morbid fear of strangers.

Yang—Male, positive energy that produces light, warmth, and fullness.

Yin—Female, negative energy. The force of darkness, cold, and emptiness.

Yoruba—The African tribe whose myths and rites are the basis of *Santeria*.

---

*These terms are defined with their traditional connotations, rather than with modern denotations (compiled over time by R. Spector).

Appendix B

Calendar: Religious Holidays That Change Dates

There are many Holy Days observed by people from many different religious heritages that do not fall on the same dates of the Julian calendar on an annual basis. Given the increasing amount of religious diversity in this country, it is imperative that consideration be given to this fact. Religious leaders of a given faith community must be contacted regarding the Julian dates of a given holiday and large meetings and other activities must not be scheduled at that time to cause conflict.

Heritage	Holiday	Approximate Date
Islam	Eid al-Fitr and Al Hisrah (New Year)	Varies
Chinese	Sending Off the Kitchen God Day	January
Islam	Laylat al-Qadr	January
Sikh	Guru Gobind Singh Ji's Birthday	January
Hindu	Makara Sakranti/Pongal	January
Chinese	New Year: Chinese, Korean, Tibetan, Vietnamese	February
Chinese	Lantern Festival	February
Baha'i	Intercalary Days	February or March
Hindu	Maha Shivaratri (Shiva's Night)	March
Christian	Shrove Monday	March
Christian	Shrove Tuesday	March
Christian	Ash Wednesday	March
Eastern Orthodox	Beginning of Lent, Eastern Orthodox Christian	March
Hindu	Holi	March
Iranian	Now Rouz	March
Chinese	Respect for Ancestors (Ch'ing-ming)	April
Islam	Muharram	April
Vietnamese	Thanh Minh (Respect for Ancestors Day)	April
Hindu	Ramanavami	April
Cambodian	New Year	April
Hindu	Vaisakhi (Solar New Year)	April
Sikh	Baisakhi (New Year)	April
Jain	Mahavir Jayanti	April
Christian	Palm Sunday	April
Jewish	Passover begins at sundown	April

Heritage	Holiday	Approximate Date
Jewish	Passover	April
Christian	Good Friday	April
Baha'i	Festival of Ridvan	April
Christian	Easter	April
Eastern Orthodox	Palm Sunday	April (a week after Christian Palm Sunday)
Christian	Easter Monday	April
Eastern Orthodox Christian	Good Friday	April (a week after Christian Good Friday)
Eastern Orthodox	Easter: Eastern Orthodox, also known as Pascha	April
Buddhist	Visakaha Day	May
Chinese	Dragon Boat Festival	June
Eastern Orthodox	Ascension Day	June
Jewish	Shavuoth begins at sundown	May or June
Christian	Pentecost	June
Islam	Maulid an-Nabi	June
Eastern Orthodox	Pentacost	June
Chinese	Seventh Night	August
Jewish	Tisha B' Av Fast Day	July or August
Hindu	Janmashtami	August
Korean	Chusok	September
Coptic Christian	Coptic New Year	September
Chinese	Midautumn Moon Festival—Chung-ch'iu	September
Jewish	Rosh Hashanah begins at sundown	September
Hindu	Durga Puja	October
Jewish	Yom Kippur begins at sundown	September or October
Jewish	Yom Kippur	October
Jewish	Sukkoth begins at sundown	October
Baha'i	Birthday of the Bab	October
Jewish	Shmini Atzeret begins at sundown	October
Jewish	Simchat Torah begins at sundown	October
Hindu	Diwali	October
Sikh	Nanak's Birthday	November
Baha'i	Birthday of Baha'u'llah	November
Islam	Ramadan	Varies

Source: Adapted from *Multicultural resource calendar.* (2000). Amherst, MA: Amherst Educational Publishing, 800-865-5549 or visit http://www.diversityresources.com. An annual calendar is available with the exact dates for the given holidays.

Appendix C

Heritage Assessment Tool

This set of questions is to be used to describe a person's—or your own—ethnic, cultural, and religious background. In performing a *heritage assessment* it is helpful to determine how deeply a person identifies with his or her traditional heritage. This tool is very useful in setting the stage for assessing and understanding a person's traditional HEALTH and ILLNESS beliefs and practices and in helping determine the community resources that will be appropriate to target for support when necessary. The greater the number of positive responses, the greater the degree to which the person may identify with his or her traditional heritage. The one exception to positive answers is the question about whether a person's name was changed. The background rationale for the development of this tool is found in Chapter 1.

1. Where was your mother born? _____

2. Where was your father born? _____

3. Where were your grandparents born? _____

    A. Your mother's mother? _____

    B. Your mother's father? _____

    C. Your father's mother? _____

    D. Your father's father? _____

4. How many brothers _____ and sisters _____ do you have?

5. What setting did you grow up in? Urban _____ Rural _____

6. What country did your parents grow up in?

    Father _____

    Mother _____

7. How old were you when you came to the United States? _____

8. How old were your parents when they came to the United States? _____

    Mother _____

    Father _____

9. When you were growing up, who lived with you?_____

_____

10. Have you maintained contact with

    A. Aunts, uncles, cousins?   (1) Yes ____ (2) No ____
    B. Brothers and sisters?   (1) Yes ____ (2) No ____
    C. Parents?   (1) Yes ____ (2) No ____
    D. Your own children?   (1) Yes ____ (2) No ____

11. Did most of your aunts, uncles, and cousins live near your home?
    (1) Yes ____
    (2) No ____

12. Approximately how often did you visit family members who lived outside of your home?
    (1) Daily ____
    (2) Weekly ____
    (3) Monthly ____
    (4) Once a year or less ____
    (5) Never ____

13. Was your original family name changed?
    (1) Yes ____
    (2) No ____

14. What is your religious preference?
    (1) Catholic ____
    (2) Jewish ____
    (3) Protestant ____ Denomination ____
    (4) Other ____
    (5) None ____

15. Is your spouse the same religion as you?
    (1) Yes ____
    (2) No ____

16. Is your spouse the same ethnic background as you?
    (1) Yes ____
    (2) No ____

17. What kind of school did you go to?
    (1) Public ____
    (2) Private ____
    (3) Parochial ____

18. As an adult, do you live in a neighborhood where the neighbors are the same religion and ethnic background as you?
    (1) Yes ____
    (2) No ____

19. Do you belong to a religious institution?
    (1) Yes ____
    (2) No ____

20. Would you describe yourself as an active member?
    (1) Yes ____
    (2) No ____
21. How often do you attend your religious institution?
    (1) More than once a week ____
    (2) Weekly ____
    (3) Monthly ____
    (4) Special holidays only ____
    (5) Never ____
22. Do you practice your religion in your home?
    (1) Yes ____ (if yes, please specify)
    (2) No ____
    (3) Praying ____
    (4) Bible reading ____
    (5) Diet ____
    (6) Celebrating religious holidays ____
23. Do you prepare foods special to your ethnic background?
    (1) Yes ____
    (2) No ____
24. Do you participate in ethnic activities?
    (1) Yes ____ (if yes, please specify)
    (2) No ____
    (3) Singing ____
    (4) Holiday celebrations ____
    (5) Dancing ____
    (6) Festivals ____
    (7) Costumes ____
    (8) Other ____
25. Are your friends from the same religious background as you?
    (1) Yes ____
    (2) No ____
26. Are your friends from the same ethnic background as you?
    (1) Yes ____
    (2) No ____
27. What is your native language other than English? _____
28. Do you speak this language?
    (1) Prefer ____
    (2) Occasionally ____
    (3) Rarely ____
29. Do you read your native language?
    (1) Yes ____
    (2) No ____

Appendix D

Quick Guide for CULTURALCARE

Preparing

- Understand your own cultural values, biases, and traditional health/HEALTH beliefs and practices.
- Acquire basic knowledge of cultural values and health/HEALTH beliefs and practices for patient groups you serve.
- Be respectful of, interested in, and understanding of other cultures without being judgmental.

Enhancing Communication

- Determine the level of fluency in English and arrange for a competent interpreter, when needed.
- Ask how the patient prefers to be addressed.
- Allow the patient to choose seating for comfortable personal space and eye contact. If the patient prefers *not* to establish eye contact, do not become upset. In many cultures, it is considered polite to avoid eye contact.
- Avoid body language and gestures that may be offensive or misunderstood.
- Speak directly and quietly to the patient, whether an interpreter is present or not.
- Choose a speech rate and style that promotes understanding and demonstrates respect for the patient.
- Avoid slang, technical jargon, and complex sentences.
- Use open-ended questions or questions phrased in several ways to obtain information.
- Determine the patient's reading ability before using written materials in the teaching process.
- Provide reading material that is easily read in the patient's native language. Do not use cartoons and cartoon characters for illustrations.

Promoting Positive Change

- Build on cultural HEALTH practices, reinforcing those that are positive and promoting change only in those that are potentially harmful.
- Check for patient understanding and acceptance of recommendations.
- Remember: Not all seeds of knowledge fall into a fertile environment to produce change. Of those that do, some will take years to germinate. Be patient and provide CULTURALCARE nursing in a culturally appropriate environment to promote positive health/HEALTH behavior.

Source: (Adapted for nursing) Schilling, B., & Brannon, E. (1986). *Cross-cultural counseling—A guide for nutrition and health counselors.* Alexandria, VA: U.S. Department of Agriculture, U.S. Department of Health and Human Services, Nutrition and Technical Services Division. Adapted with permission.

Appendix E

Data Resources

Countless invaluable resources are available in both the public and private sectors.

1. The United States Census
2. United States Citizenship and Immigration Services
3. Office for Civil Rights
4. National Center for Health Statistics—*Healthy People 2010*
5. National Health Statistics
6. Health Resources and Services Administration (HRSA)
7. The Office of Minority Health
8. Complementary and alternative medicine
9. Specific health-related sites
10. Consumer information
11. Private sector

It is important to note that the URLs change; however, the new addresses are usually linked to the old site.

The United States Census

http://www.census.gov

This page provides links to census information at national, state, county, and local levels.

It also has statistics related to income, housing, and so forth.

Homeland Security

This agency has responsibility for information regarding immigration, commerce and trade, and emergency preparedness.

http://www.dhs.gov/index.shtm

United States Citizenship and Immigration Services

http://www.uscis.gov/portal/site/uscis

This site has information regarding citizenship application process.

http://www.usimmigrationsupport.org/?NS_cid=1

This site has helpful information for immigrants.

Office for Civil Rights

The Office for Civil Rights is located within the U.S. Department of Health and Human Services and is responsible for enforcing the nondiscrimination requirements of Title VI of the Civil Rights Act of 1964.

http://www.hhs.gov/ocr/discrimrace.html

National Center for Health Statistics—*Healthy People 2010*

The purpose of the National Center for Health Statistics is to monitor the nation's health. The goals have been set for health status for 2010 and the *Healthy People 2010 Mid-course Review* is now available online. This publication assesses progress toward achieving the *Healthy People 2010* goals and objectives through the first half of the decade.

http://www.cdc.gov/nchs/hphome.htm

National Health Statistics

The database Health, United States, is available from this source annually and has current information on a myriad of population- and health-related issues.

http://www.cdc.gov/nchs/Default.htm

Health Resources and Services Administration (HRSA)

This site has information regarding health professions and the health care system.

http://www.hrsa.gov

Other government health-related resources include the following:

U.S. Department of Health and Human Services

This agency's goal is "improving the health, safety, and well-being of America."

http://www.dhhs.gov

Center for Medicare & Medicaid Services

The mission of this agency is to ensure effective, up-to-date health care coverage and to promote quality care for beneficiaries.

http://www.cms.hhs.gov

Center for Disease Control and Prevention

This site provides links to countless credible health information resources.

http://www.cdc.gov

CDC's National Center for Chronic Disease Prevention and Health Promotion

http://www.cdc.gov/nccdphp/

National Information Center on Health Services Research and Health Care Technology (NICHSR)

The purpose of this agency is improving the collection, storage, analysis, retrieval, and dissemination of health services research.

http://www.nlm.nih.gov/nichsr

Healthfinder

Since 1997, healthfinder.gov has been recognized as a key resource for finding the best government and nonprofit health and human services information on the Internet. There are links to carefully selected information and Web sites from over 1,500 health-related organizations.

http://www.healthfinder.gov

The Office of Minority Health

National Center on Minority Health and Health Disparities

The mission of the National Center on Minority Health and Health Disparities (NCMHD) is to promote minority health and to lead, coordinate, support, and assess the NIH effort to reduce and ultimately eliminate health disparities. In this effort NCMHD will conduct and support basic, clinical, social, and behavioral research, promote research infrastructure and training, and foster emerging programs.

http://www.ncmhd.nih.gov

Complementary and Alternative Medicine

The National Center for Complementary and Alternative Medicine (NCCAM) is the federal government's lead agency for scientific research on complementary and alternative medicine (CAM). The mission of NCCAM is to

▓ Explore complementary and alternative healing practices in the context of rigorous science

▓ Train complementary and alternative medicine researchers

▓ Disseminate authoritative information to the public and professionals

http://nccam.nih.gov/

Specific Health-Related Sites—Public Resources

Aging

National Aging Information Center

The bibliographic database is managed by the Center for Communication and Consumer Services (CCCS). It contains references to program- and policy-related materials on aging not referenced in any other computer system or print resource. The database is intended to serve the State Units on Aging, Area Agencies on Aging, national aging organizations, aging services providers, legislators at all levels, policymakers, and the general public.

http://www.aoa.gov/naic

National Institute on Aging

http://www.nih.gov/nia/health

AIDS/HIV

AIDSinfo

AIDS*info* is a U.S. Department of Health and Human Services (DHHS) project that offers the latest federally approved information on HIV/AIDS clinical research, treatment and prevention, and medical practice guidelines for people living with HIV/AIDS, their families and friends, health care providers, scientists, and researchers.

http://www.hivatis.org

Diabetes

National Diabetes Surveillance System

The CDC Diabetes Surveillance System collects, analyzes, and disseminates data on diabetes and its complications. This public health surveillance (disease tracking) of diabetes is critical to

- Increase recognition of the disease
- Identify high-risk groups
- Develop strategies to reduce the economic and human cost of this disease
- Formulate health care policy
- Evaluate progress in disease prevention and control

The current Diabetes Surveillance System updates data from previous reports and will also contain new surveillance topics.

http://www.cdc.gov/diabetes/statistics/index.htm#prevalence

National Diabetes Education Program

http://ndep.nih.gov

Cancer

National Cancer Institute

This site contains links to a myriad of information regarding all aspects of cancer from diagnosis through various treatment modalities and options.

http://www.cancer.gov/

Heart Disease and Heart Health

National Heart, Lung, and Blood Institute (NHLBI) Health Information Center

The National Heart, Lung, and Blood Institute provides global leadership for a research, training, and education program to promote the prevention and treatment of heart, lung, and blood diseases and fulfilling lives.

http://www.nhlbi.nih.gov

Immunization

The National Immunization Program (NIP): Centers for Disease Control and Prevention

http://www.cdc.gov/vaccines

Injury Prevention

National Center for Injury Prevention and Control (NCIPC)

http://www.cdc.gov/ncipc

Lead Poisoning

National Lead Information Center

This site provides information about lead and lead hazards and provides some simple steps to protect the family.

http://www.epa.gov/lead/

Rural Health

Rural Information Center Health Service (RICHS)

Rural Health Funding Sources: National Foundations

This guide represents private and nonprofit foundations that fund programs related to rural health.

http://www.nal.usda.gov/ric/ricpubs/foundat.htm

San Francisco State University

Unnatural Causes: Is Inequality Making Us Sick?

An excellent film series about what are the sources of sickness in 2008.

http://www.pbs.org/unnaturalcauses/Or 1-877-7495.

Consumer Information Center

The Federal Citizen Information Center

USA.gov is the official portal to all government information, services, and transactions. This site pulls together more than 180 million federal, state, and local government Web pages. Here, citizens can get easy-to-understand information and services from the government 24 hours a day, 7 days a week. They can also use an e-mail form to send questions and comments in English and Spanish for a response within 2 business days.

http://www.usa.gov

Private Sector

There are countless agencies available in this sector, including numerous networks. The following Web page is a well-developed resource to link to the agencies.

http://www.healthpowerforminorities.org/resources/national.cfm

(The URLs of all sites listed have been checked and are current as of this publishing date.)

Johnson and Johnson Diabetes Institute

Addresses the shortage in diabetes specific training and offers training
http://www.jjdi.us/

Bibliography

Abraham, L. K. (1993). *Mama might be better off dead: The failure of health care in urban America*. Chicago: University of Chicago Press.

Abrahams, P. (1954). *Tell freedom: Memories of Africa*. New York: Knopf.

Achebe, C. (1987). *Anthills of Savannah*. New York: Anchor Press/Doubleday.

Achebe, C. (1959). *Things fall apart*. Greenwich, CT: Fawcett Crest.

Achterberg, J., Dossey, B., & Kolkmeier, L. (1994). *Rituals of healing: Using imagery for health and wellness*. New York: Bantam Books.

Aday, L. A. (1993). *At risk in America—The health and health care needs of vulnerable populations in the United States*. San Francisco: Jossey-Bass.

Aiken, L. G. (1981). *Health policy and nursing practice*. New York: McGraw-Hill.

Aiken, R. (1980). *Mexican folk tales from the borderland*. Dallas, TX: Southern Methodist University Press.

Albrecht, G. L., & Higgens, P. C. (Eds.). (1979). *Health, illness, and medicine*. Chicago: Rand McNally.

Alcott, W. A. (1839). *The house I live in; or the human body*. Boston, MA: George W. Light.

Allende, I. (1993). *The house of the spirits*. New York: Bantam Books.

Allison, D. (1992). *Bastard out of Carolina*. New York: Plume.

Allport, G. W. (1958). *The nature of prejudice* (abridged). Garden City, NY: Doubleday.

Alvarez, H. R. (1975). *Health without boundaries*. Mexico: United States–Mexico Border Public Health Association.

Alvarez, J. (1992). *How the Garcia girls lost their accents*. New York: Plume.

Ameer Ali, S. (1922, 1978). *The spirit of Islam*. Delhi, India: IDARAH-I-ADABIYAT-I-DELLI.

American Nurses' Association. (1979, June 9–10). *A strategy for change*. Papers presented at the conference of the Commission on Human Rights, Albuquerque, NM.

American Psychiatric Association. (1994). *Diagnostic and statistical manual of mental disorders* (4th ed.). Washington, DC: Author.

Anderson, D. M. (1995). *Maasai people of cattle*. San Francisco: Chronicle Books.

Anderson, E. T., & McFarlane, J. M. (1988). *Community as client*. Philadelphia, PA: J. B. Lippincott.

Anderson, J. Q. (1970). *Texas folk medicine*. Austin, TX: Encino Press.

Andrade, S. J. (1978). *Chicano mental health: The case of cristal*. Austin: Hogg Foundation for Mental Health.

Andrews, E. D. (1953). *The people called Shakers*. New York: Dover.

Andrews, M. M., & Boyle, J. S. (1995). *Transcultural concepts in nursing care* (2nd ed.). Philadelphia, PA: J. B. Lippincott.

Angelou, M. (1970). *I know why the caged bird sings*. New York: Random House.

Annas, G. J. (1975). *The rights of hospital patients*. New York: Avon.

Appelfeld, A. (1990). *The healer*. New York: Grove Weidenfeld.

Apple, D. (Ed.). (1960). *Sociological studies of health and sickness: A source book for the health professions*. New York: McGraw-Hill, Blakiston Division.

Archer, S. E., & Fleshman, R. P. (1985). *Community health nursing* (3rd ed.). Monterey, CA: Wadsworth.

Armstrong, D., & Armstrong, E. M. (1991). *The great American medicine show.* New York: Prentice Hall.

Arnold, M. G., & Rosenbaum, G. (1973). *The crime of poverty.* Skokie, IL: National Textbook Co.

Ashely, J. (1976). *Hospitals, paternalism, and the role of the nurse.* New York: Teachers College Press.

Aurand, A. M., Jr. (n.d.). *The realness of witchcraft in America.* Lancaster, PA: Aurand Press.

Ausubel, N. (1964). *The book of Jewish knowledge.* New York: Crown.

Bahti, T. (1974). *Southwestern Indian ceremonials.* Las Vegas: KC Publications.

Bahti, T. (1975). *Southwestern Indian tribes.* Las Vegas: KC Publications.

Bakan, D. (1968). *Disease, pain, and sacrifice: Toward a psychology of suffering.* Chicago: University of Chicago Press.

Baker, G. C. (1994). *Planning and organizing for multicultural instruction* (2nd ed.). Menlo Park, CA: Addison-Wesley.

Balch, J. F., & Balch, P. A. (1990). *Prescription for nutritional healing.* Garden City Park, NY: Avery.

Baldwin, R. (1986). *The healers.* Huntington, IN: Our Sunday Visitor.

Banks, J. A. (Ed.). (1973). *Teaching ethnic studies.* Washington, DC: National Council for Social Studies.

Bannerman, R. H., Burton, J., & Wen-Chieh, C. (1983). *Traditional medicine and health care coverage.* Geneva: World Health Organization.

Barden, T. E. (Ed.). (1991). *Virginia folk legends.* Charlottesville: University Press of Virginia.

Bauwens, E. F. (1979). *The anthropology of health.* St. Louis, MO: C. V. Mosby.

Bear, S., & Bear, W. (1996). *The medicine wheel.* New York: Fireside.

Beaudoin, T. (1998). *Virtual Faith: The irreverent spiritual quest of generation X.* San Francisco: Jossey Bass.

Becerra, R. M., & Shaw, D. (1984). *The elderly Hispanic: A research and reference guide.* Lanham, MD: University Press of America.

Becker, M. H. (1974). *The health belief model and personal health behavior.* Thorofare, NJ: Slack.

Beimler, R. R. (1991). *The days of the dead.* San Francisco: Collins Publishers.

Belgium, D. (Ed.). (1967). *Religion and medicine.* Ames: Iowa State University Press.

Ben-Amos, D., & Mintz, J. R. (1970). *In praise of the Baal Shem Tov.* New York: Shocken Books.

Benedict, R. (1946). *Patterns of culture.* New York: Penguin Books.

Benjamin, G. G. (1910, reprint 1974). *The Germans in Texas.* Austin: Jenkins.

Bennett, C. I. (1990). *Comprehensive multicultural education* (2nd ed.). Boston: Allyn and Bacon.

Benson, H. (1996). *Timeless healing.* New York: Scribner.

Berg, D. J. (Ed.). (1986). *Homestead hints.* Berkeley, CA: Ten Speed Press.

Berg, P. S. (Ed.). (1977). *An entrance to the tree of life.* Jerusalem, Israel: Research Center for Kabbalah.

Berman, E. (1976). *The solid gold stethoscope.* New York: Macmillan Co.

Bermann, E. (1973). *Scapegoat.* Ann Arbor: University of Michigan Press.

Bernardo, A. (n.d.). *Lourdes: Then and now.* Trans. Rand, P. T. Lourdes, France: Etablissements Estrade.

Bernardo, S. (1981). *The ethnic almanac.* Garden City, NY: Doubleday.

Berwick, D. M., Godfrey, A. B., & Roessner, J. (1990). *Curing health care.* San Francisco: Jossey-Bass.

Bienvenue, R. M., & Goldstein, J. E. (1979). *Ethnicity and ethnic relations in Canada* (2nd ed.). Toronto: Butterworths.

Birnbaum, P. (1988). *Encyclopedia of Jewish concepts.* New York: Hebrew.

Bishop, G. (1967). *Faith healing: God or fraud?* Los Angeles: Shervourne Press.

Bohannan, P. (1992). *We, the alien.* Prospect Heights, IL: Waveland Press, Inc.

Boney, W. (1939). *The French Canadians today.* London: J. M. Dent and Sons.

Bonfanti, L. (1974). *Biographies and legends of the New England Indians,* Vol. 4. Wakefield, MA: Pride.

Bonfanti, L. (1980). *Strange beliefs, customs, and superstitions of New England.* Wakefield, MA: Pride.

Bottomore, T. B. (1968). *Classes in modern society.* New York: Vintage Books.

Bowen, E. S. (1964). *Return to laughter.* Garden City, NY: Doubleday.

Bowker, J. (1991). *The meanings of death.* Cambridge: Cambridge University Press.

Boyd, D. (1974). *Rolling thunder.* New York: Random House.

Boyle, J. S., & Andrews, M. M. (1995). *Transcultural concepts in nursing care* (2nd ed.). Philadelphia, PA: J. B. Lippincott.

Bracq, J. C. (1924). *The evolution of French Canada.* New York: Macmillan.

Bradley, C. J. (1980). "Characteristics of Women and Infants Attended by Lay Midwives in Texas, 1971: A Case Comparison Study." Master's thesis, University of Texas Health Science Center at Houston, School of Public Health.

Branch, M. F., & Paxton, P. P. (1976). *Providing safe nursing care for ethnic people of color.* New York: Appleton-Century-Crofts.

Brand, J. (1978). *The life and death of Anna Mae Aquash.* Toronto: James Lorimer.

Brandon, G. (1997). *Santeria: From Africa to the New World.* Bloomington: University of Indiana Press.

Brink, J., & Keen, L. (1979). *Feverfew.* London: Century.

Brink, P. J. (Ed.). (1976). *Transcultural nursing: A book of readings.* Englewood Cliffs, NJ: Prentice Hall.

Brown, D. (1970). *Bury my heart at Wounded Knee.* New York: Holt, Rinehart & Winston.

Brown, D. (1980). *Creek Mary's blood.* New York: Holt, Rinehart & Winston.

Browne, G., Howard, J., & Pitts, M. (1985). *Culture and children.* Austin: University of Texas Press.

Browne, K., & Freeling, P. (1967). *The doctor–patient relationship.* Edinburgh: E & S Livingstone.

Brownlee, A. T. (1979). *Community, culture, and care: A cross cultural guide for healthworkers.* St. Louis, MO: C. V. Mosby.

Bruchac, J. (1985). *Iroquois stories heroes and heroines monsters and magic.* Freedom, CA: Crossing Press.

Bryant, C. A. (1985). *The cultural feast: An introduction to food and society.* St. Paul, MN: West.

Buchman, D. D. (1979). *Herbal medicine: The natural way to get well and stay well.* New York: Gramercy.

Budge, E. A. W. (1978). *Amulets and superstitions.* New York: Dover.

Bullough, B., & Bullough, V. L. (1972). *Poverty, ethnic identity, and health care.* New York: Appleton-Century-Crofts.

Bullough, V. L., & Bullough, B. (1982). *Health care for other Americans.* New York: Appleton-Century-Crofts.

Butler, H. (1967). *Doctor gringo.* New York: Rand McNally.

Buxton, J. (1973). *Religion and healing in Mandari.* Oxford: Clarendon Press.

Cafferty, P. S. J., Chiswick, B. R., Greeley, A. M., et al. (1983). *The dilemma of American immigration: Beyond the golden door.* New Brunswick, NJ: Transaction Books.

Cahill, R. E. (1990). *Olde New England's curious customs and cures.* Salem, MA: Old Saltbox Publishing House.

Cahill, R. E. (1990). *Strange superstitions.* Salem, MA: Old Saltbox Publishing House.

Calhoun, M. (1976). *Medicine show.* New York: Harper and Row.

Califano, J. (1994). *Radical surgery.* New York: Random House.

Campos, E. (1955). *Medicina popular: Supersticione credios e meizinhas* (2nd ed.). Rio de Janeiro: Livraria-Editora da Casa.

Candill, H. M. (1962). *Night comes to the Cumberlands.* Boston: Little, Brown.

Carnegie, M. E. (1987). *The path we tread: Blacks in nursing 1854–1984.* Philadelphia, PA: J. B. Lippincott.

Carson, V. B. (Ed.). (1989). *Spiritual dimensions of nursing practice.* Philadelphia, PA: W. B. Saunders.

Catlin, G. (1993). *North American Indian portfolios.* New York: Abbeville.

Chafets, Z. (1990). *Devil's night and other tales of Detroit.* New York: Vintage Books.

Chan, L. S., McCandless, R., Portnoy, B., et al. (1987). *Maternal and child health on the U.S.–Mexico border.* Austin: The University of Texas.

Chavira, L. (1975). *Curanderismo: An optional health-care system.* Edinburg, TX: Pan American University.

Chenault, L. R. (1938). *The Puerto Rican migrant in New York City.* New York: Columbia University Press.

Chiba, R. (1966). *The seven lucky gods of Japan.* Rutland, VT: Charles E. Tuttle Co.

Choron, J. (1964). *Death and modern man.* New York: Collier Books.

Chun, M. N. (1986). *Hawaiian medicine book.* Honolulu: Bess Press.

Chute, C. (1985). *The beans of Egypt, Maine.* New York: Ticknor & Fields.

Clark, A. (1978). *Culture, childbearing health professionals.* Philadelphia, PA: F. A. Davis.

Clark, A. L. (1981). *Culture and child rearing.* Philadelphia, PA: F. A. Davis.

Clark, M. (1959). *Health in the Mexican-American culture: A community study.* Berkeley: University of California Press.

Comas-Diaz, L., & Griffith, E. E. H. (1988). *Clinical guidelines in cross-cultural mental health.* New York: Wiley.

Committee on Medical Care Teaching (Eds.). (1958). *Readings in medical care.* Chapel Hill: University of North Carolina Press.

Conde, M. I. (1992). *Tituba, black witch of Salem.* New York: Ballantine Books.

Conway, M. (1974). *Rise gonna rise.* New York: Anchor Books.

Corish, J. L. (1923). *Health knowledge,* Vol. 1. New York: Domestic Health Society.

Cornacchia, H. J. (1976). *Consumer health.* St. Louis, MO: C. V. Mosby.

Corum, A. K. (1985). *Folk remedies from Hawai'i.* Honolulu: Bess Press.

Council of Churches. (1995). *Knowing my neighbor, religious beliefs and traditions at times of illness and death.* Springfield, MA: Visiting Nurse Hospice of Pioneer Valley.

Council on Cultural Diversity in Nursing Practice. (1994). *Proceedings of the Invitational Meeting on Multicultural Issues in the Nursing Workforce and Workplace.* Washington, DC: American Nurses Association.

Cowan, N. M., & Cowan, R. S. (1989). *Our parents' lives.* New York: Basic Books.

Cramer, M. E. (1923). *Divine science and healing*. Denver: Colorado College of Divine Science.

Crichton, M. (1970). *Five patients*. New York: Alfred A. Knopf.

Crispino, J. A. (1980). *Assimilation of ethnic groups: The Italian case*. Newark, NJ: New Jersey Center for Migration.

Cross, T. (1994). Understanding family resiliency from a relational worldview. In *Resiliency in families: Racial and ethnic minority families in America*. Madison: University of Wisconsin–Madison.

Crow Dog, L., & Erdoes, R. (1996). *Crow Dog*. San Francisco: Harper.

Culpeper, N. (1889). *Culpeper's complete herbal*. London: W. Foulsham.

Curry, M. A., project director. (1987). *Access to prenatal care: Key to preventing low birth weight*. Kansas City, MO: American Nurses Association.

Curtis, E. (1993). *Native American wisdom*. Philadelphia, PA: Running Press.

Cutter, C. (1850). *First book on anatomy, physiology, and hygiene, for grammar schools and families*. Boston, MA: Benjamin B. Mussey.

Danforth, L. M. (1982). *The death rituals of rural Greece*. Princeton, NJ: Princeton University Press.

Davis, F. (Ed.). (1966). *The nursing profession: Five sociological essays*. New York: Wiley.

Davis, R. (1998). *American voudou: Journey into a hidden world*. Denton, TX: University of North Texas Press.

DeBella, S., Martin, L., & Siddall, S. (1986). *Nurses' role in health care planning*. Norwalk, CT: Appleton-Century-Crofts.

De Castro, J. (1967). *The black book of hunger*. Boston, MA: Beacon Press.

Delaney, J., Lupton, M. J., & Toth, E. (1988). *The curse: A cultural history of menstruation*. Chicago: University of Chicago Press.

Deller, B., Hicks, D., & MacDonald, G., coordinators. (1979). *Stone boats and lone stars*. Hyde Park, Ontario: Middlesex County Board of Education.

Deloria, V. Jr. (1969). *Custer died for our sins: An Indian manifesto*. New York: Avon Books.

DeLys, C. (1948). *A treasury of American superstitions*. New York: Philosophical Library.

Densmore, F. (1974). *How Indians use wild plants for food, medicine, and crafts*. New York: Dover.

Deren, M. (1953). *Divine horseman: The living gods of Haiti*. New York: McPherson.

Dey, C. (1982). *The magic candle*. Bronx, NY: Original Publications.

Dickerson, J. (1998). *Dixie's dirty secret*. Armonk, NY: Sharpe.

Dickison, R. (Ed.). (1987). *Causes, cures, sense, and nonsense*. Sacramento, CA: Bishop Publishing Co.

Dinnerstein, L., & Reimers, D. M. (1988). *Ethnic Americans* (3rd ed.). New York: Harper & Row.

Dioszegi, V. (1996). *Folk beliefs and shamanistic practices in Siberia*. Budapest: Akademiai Kiado.

Doane, N. L. (1985). *Indian doctor book*. Charlotte, NC: Aerial.

Doka, K. J., & Morgan, J. D. (Eds.). (1993). *Death and spirituality*. Amityville, NY: Baywood.

Donegan, J. B. (1978). *Women and men midwives: Medicine, morality, and misogyny in early America*. Westport, CT: Greenwood Press.

Donin, H. H. (1972). *To be a Jew*. New York: Basic Books.

Dorris, M. (1989). *The broken cord*. New York: Harper & Row.

Dorson, R. H. D. (Ed.). (1972). *Folklore and folklife*. Chicago: University of Chicago Press.

Dossey, L. (1993). *Healing words*. San Francisco: Harper.

Dresser, N. (1993). Our Own Stories: *Cross-cultural communication practice.* White Plains, NY: Longman.

Dresser, N. (1999). *Multicultural celebrations.* New York: Three Rivers Press.

Dresser, N. (1996). *Multicultural manners.* New York: Wiley.

Dubos, R. (1968). *Man, medicine and environment.* New York: Mentor.

Dubos, R. (1961). *Mirage of health.* Garden City, NY: Anchor Books, Doubleday and Co.

Dubos, R. J. (1965). *Man adapting.* New Haven, CT: Yale University Press.

Dworaczyk, E. J. (1979). *The first Polish colonies of America in Texas.* San Antonio, TX: The Naylor Company.

Eck, D. L. (1998). *World religions in Boston* (2nd ed.). Cambridge: Harvard University Press.

Egan, M. (1991). *Milagros.* Santa Fe: Museum of New Mexico Press.

Ehrenreich, B., & Ehrenreich, J. (1970). *The American health empire: Power, profits, and politics.* New York: Random House, Vintage Books.

Ehrenreich, B., & English, D. (1973). *Witches, midwives, and nurses: A history of women healers* (2nd ed.). Old Westbury, NY: Feminist Press.

Ehrlich, P. R. (1979). *The golden door: International migration, Mexico and the United States.* New York: Wideview Books.

Eichler, L. (1923). *The customs of mankind.* Garden City, NY: Doubleday, Page.

Eisenberg, D. (1985). *Encounters with Qi.* New York: W. W. Norton.

Eisinger, P. K. (1998). *Toward an end to hunger in America.* Washington, DC: Brookings Institution.

Eliade, M., & Couliano, I. P. (1991). *The Eliade guide to world religions.* San Francisco: Harper.

Elling, R. H. (1977). *Socio-cultural influences on health and health care.* New York: Springer.

Elworthy, R. T. (1958). *The evil eye: The origins and practices of superstition.*

New York: Julian Press. (Originally published by John Murray, London, 1915.)

Epstein, C. (1974). *Effective interaction in contemporary nursing.* Englewood Cliffs, NJ: Prentice Hall.

Evans, E. F. (1881). *The divine law of cure.* Boston, MA: H. H. Carter.

Fadiman, A. (1997). *The spirit catches you and you fall down.* New York: Farrar, Straus and Giroux.

Farge, E. J. (1975). *La vida Chicana: Health care attitudes and behaviors of Houston Chicanos.* San Francisco: R and E Research Associates.

Feagin, J. R. (1975). *Subordinating the poor: Welfare and American beliefs.* Englewood Cliffs, NJ: Prentice Hall.

Feagin, J. R., & Feagin, C. B. (1978). *Discrimination American style.* Englewood Cliffs, NJ: Prentice Hall.

Feldman, D. M. (1986). *Health and medicine in the Jewish tradition.* New York: Crossroads.

Finney, J. C. (Ed.). (1969). *Culture change, mental health, and poverty.* New York: Simon and Schuster.

Fleming, A. S., chairman, U.S. Commission on Civil Rights. (1980). *The tarnished golden door: Civil rights issues on immigration.* Washington, DC: Government Printing Office.

Flores-Pena, Y., & Evanchuk, R. J. (1994). *Santeria garments and altars.* Jackson: University of Mississippi Press.

Fonseca, I. (1995). *Bury me standing: The gypsies and their journey.* New York: Vintage.

Forbes, T. R. (1966). *The midwife and the witch.* New Haven, CT: Yale University Press.

Ford, P. S. (1971). *The healing trinity: Prescriptions for body, mind, and spirit.* New York: Harper & Row.

Fox, M. (2001). *One river, many wells.* New York: Tarcher/Putnam.

Foy, F. A. (Ed.). (1980). *Catholic Almanac.* Huntington, IN: Our Sunday Visitor.

Francis, P., Jr. (1994). *Beads of the world*. Atglen, PA: Schiffer.

Frankel, E., & Teutsch, B. P. (1992). *The encyclopedia of Jewish symbols*. Northvale, NJ: Jason Aronson, Inc.

Frazer, J. G. (1923). *Folklore in the Old Testament*. New York: Tudor Publishing.

Freedman, L. (1969). *Public housing: The politics of poverty*. New York: Holt, Rinehart & Winston.

Freeman, H., Levine, S., & Reeder, L. G. (Eds.). (1972). *Handbook of medical sociology* (2nd ed.). Englewood Cliffs, NJ: Prentice Hall.

Freidson, E. (1971). *Profession of medicine*. New York: Dodd, Mead.

Freire, P. (1970). *Pedagogy of the oppressed*. Trans. M. B. Ramos. New York: Seabury Press.

Friedman, M., & Friedland, G. W. (1998). *Medicine's ten greatest discoveries*. New Haven, CT: Yale University Press.

Frost, M. (n.d.). *The Shaker story*. Canterbury, NH: Canterbury Shakers.

Fuentes, C. (1985). *The old gringo*. New York: Farrar, Straus and Giroux.

Fuller, J. G. (1974). *Arigo: Surgeon of the rusty knife*. New York: Pocket Books.

Galloway, M. R. U. (Ed.). (1990). *Aunt Mary, tell me a story*. Cherokee, NC: Cherokee Communications.

Gambino, R. (1974). *Blood of my blood: The dilemma of Italian-Americans*. Garden City, NY: Doubleday.

Gans, H. J. (1962). *The urban villagers*. New York: Free Press.

Garcia, C. (1992). *Dreaming in Cuban*. New York: Ballantine Books.

Garner, J. (1976). *Healing yourself* (6th ed.). Vashon, WA: Crossing Press.

Gaver, J. R. (1972). *Sickle cell disease*. New York: Lancer Books.

Gaw, A. (Ed.). (1982). *Cross-cultural psychiatry*. Boston, MA: John Wright.

Geissler, E. M. (1998). *Pocket guide cultural assessment* (2nd ed.). St. Louis, MO: Mosby.

Gelfond, D. E., & Kutzik, A. (Eds.). (1979). *Ethnicity and aging: Theory, research and policy*. New York: Springer.

Genovese, E. D. (1972). *Roll, Jordan, Roll*. New York: Vintage Books.

Gibbs, J. T., Huang, L. N., Nagata, D. K., et al. (1988). *Children of Color*. San Francisco: Jossey-Bass.

Gibbs, T. (1996). *A guide to ethnic health collections in the United States*. Westport, CT.: Greenwood.

Giger, J. N., & Davidhizar, R. E. (1995). *Transcultural nursing assessment and intervention* (2nd ed.). St. Louis: Mosby.

Giordano, J., & Giordano, G. P. (1977). *The Ethno-Cultural factor in mental health*. New York: New York Institute of Pluralism and Group Identity.

Glazer, N., & Moynihan, D. (Eds.). (1975). *Ethnicity: Theory and experience*. Cambridge: Harvard University Press.

Goldberg B. (1993). *Alternative medicine: The definitive guide*. Puyallup, WA: Future Medicine.

Gonzalez-Wippler, M. (1987). *Santeria: African magic in Latin America*. Bronx, NY: Original Publications.

Gonzalez-Wippler, M. (1985). *Tales of the Orishas*. New York: Original Publications.

Gonzalez-Wippler, M. (1982). *The Santeria experience*. Bronx, NY: Original Publications.

Gordon, A. F., & Kahan, L. (1976). *The tribal beads: A handbook of African trade beads*. New York: Tribal Arts Gallery.

Gordon, D. M. (1972). *Theories of poverty and underemployment*. Lexington, MA: D. C. Heath.

Gordon, F. (1966). *Role theory and illness*. New Haven, CT: College and University Press.

Goswami, S. D. (1983). *Prabhupada: He built a house in which the whole world can live*. Los Angeles: The Bhaktivedanta Book Trust.

Grant, G. (1994). *Obake: Ghost stories in Hawaii.* Honolulu: Mutual.

Gray, K. (1992). *Passport to understanding.* Denver: Center for Teaching International Relations.

Greeley, A. M. (1975). *The Irish Americans.* New York: Harper & Row.

Greeley, A. M. (1975). *Why can't they be like us? America's white ethnic groups.* New York: E. P. Dutton.

Grier, W. H., & Cobbs, P. M. (1968). *Black rage.* New York: Bantam Books.

Griffin, J. H. (1960). *Black like me.* New York: Signet.

Gruber R. (1987). *Rescue: The exodus of the Ethiopian Jews.* New York: Atheneum.

Gutman, H. G. (1976). *The black family in slavery and freedom, 1750–1925.* New York: Pantheon Books.

Gutmanis, J. (1994). *Kahuna La'au Lapa'au.* Aiea, Hawaii: Island Heritage Press.

Hailey, A. (1984). *Strong medicine.* Garden City, NY: Doubleday.

Hailey, A. (1976). *Roots.* Garden City, NY: Doubleday.

Hallam, E. (1994). *Saints.* New York: Simon & Schuster.

Hammerschlag, C. A. (1988). *The dancing healers.* San Francisco: Harper & Row.

Hand, W. D. (1973). *American folk medicine: A symposium.* Berkeley: University of California Press.

Hand, W. D. (1980). *Magical medicine.* Berkeley: University of California Press.

Harney, R. F., & Troper, H. (1975). *Immigrants: A portrait of urban experience 1890–1930.* Toronto: Van Nostrand Reinhold.

Harrington, C., & Estes, C. L. (1994). *Health policy and nursing.* Boston: Jones & Bartlett.

Harris, L. (1985). *Holy days: The world of a Hasidic family.* New York: Summit Books.

Harwood, A. (1971). "The Hot-Cold Theory of Disease: Implications for Treatment of Puerto Rican Patients," *Journal of the American Medical Asssociation, 216,* 1154–1155.

Harwood, A. (1981). (Ed.). *Ethnicity and medical care.* Cambridge, MA: Harvard University Press.

Haskins, J. (1978). *Voodoo and hoodoo.* Bronx, NY: Original Publications.

Hauptman, L. M., & Wherry, J. D. (1990). *The Pequots in southern New England: The fall and rise of an American Indian nation.* Norman: University of Oklahoma Press.

Hawkins, J. B. W., & Higgins, L. P. (1983). *Nursing and the health care delivery system.* New York: Tiresias Press.

Hecker, M. (1979). *Ethnic American, 1970–1977.* Dobbs Ferry, NY: Oceana.

Henderson, G., & Primeaux, M. (Eds.). (1981). *Transcultural health care.* Menlo Park, CA: Addison-Wesley.

Hennessee, O. M. (1989). *Aloe: Myth-magic medicine.* Lawton, OK: Universal Graphics.

Hernandez, C. A., Haug, M. J., & Wagner, N. N. (1976). *Chicanos' social and psychological perspectives.* St. Louis, MO: C. V. Mosby.

Herzlich, C. (1973). *Health and illness: A social psychological analysis.* Trans. D. Graham. New York: Academic Press.

Hiatt, H. H. (1987). *America's health in the balance: Choice or chance?* New York: Harper & Row.

Hickel, W. J. (1972). *Who owns America?* New York: Paperback Library.

Himmelstein, D. U., & Woolhandler, S. (1994). *The national health program book: A source guide for advocates.* Monroe, ME: Common Courage Press.

Hirsch, E. D. (1987). *Cultural literacy: What every American needs to know.* Boston, MA: Houghton Mifflin.

Hongo, F. M. (Gen. Ed.). (1985). *Japanese American journey: The story of a people*. San Mateo, CA: Japanese American Curriculum Project.

Honychurch, P. N. (1980). *Caribbean wild plants and their uses*. London: Macmillan.

Howard, M. (1980). *Candle burning* (2nd ed.). Weingborough, Northamptonshire, England: Aquarian Press.

Howe, I. (1976). *World of our fathers*. New York: Harcourt Brace Jovanovich.

Hufford, D. J. (1984). *American healing systems: An introduction and exploration*. Conference booklet. Philadelphia: University of Pennsylvania.

Hughes, H. S. (1953). *The United States and Italy*. Cambridge, MA: Harvard University Press.

Hughes, L., & Bontemps, A. (Eds.). (1958). *The Book of negro folklore*. New York: Dodd, Mead.

Hunter, J. D. (1994). *Before the shooting begins: Searching for democracy in America's culture war*. New York: Free Press.

Hunter, J. D. (1991). *Culture wars: The struggle to define America*. New York: Basic Books.

Hurmence, B. (Ed.). (1984). *My folks don't want me to talk about slavery*. Winston-Salem, NC: John F. Blair.

Hutchens, A. R. (1973). *Indian herbalogy of North America*. Windsor, Ontario: Meico.

Hutton, J. B. (1975). *The healing power*. London: Leslie Frewin.

Illich, I. (1975). *Medical nemesis: The expropriation of health*. London: Marion Bogars.

Illich, I., Zola, I. K., McKnight, J., et al. (1977). *Disabling professions*. Salem, NH: Boyars.

Iorizzo, L. J. (1980). *Italian immigration and the impact of the Padrone System*. New York: Arno Press.

Jackson, J. S., Chatters, L. M., & Taylor, R. J. (1993). *Aging in black America*. Newbury Park, CA: Sage.

Jaco, E. G. (Ed.). (1958). *Patients, physicians, and illness: Sourcebook in behavioral science and medicine*. Glencoe, IL: Free Press.

Jacobs, H. A. (1988). *Incidents in the life of a slave girl*. London: Oxford University Press.

Jacobs, L. (Ed.). (1990). *The Jewish mystics*. London: Kyle Cathie.

Jangl, A. M., & Jangl, J. F. (1987). *Ancient legends of healing herbs*. Coeur d'Alene, ID: Prisma Press.

Jarvis, D. C. (1958). *Folk medicine: A Vermont doctor's guide to good health*. New York: Henry Holt.

Jennings, P., & Brewater, T. (1998). *The twentieth century*. New York: Doubleday.

Jilek, W. G. (1992). *Indian healing: Shamanic ceremonialism in the Pacific Northwest today*. Blaine, WA: Hancock House.

Johnson, C. J., & McGee, M. G. (Eds.). (1991). *How different religions view death and afterlife*. Philadelphia, PA: Charles Press.

Johnson, C. L. (1985). *Growing up and growing old in Italian-American families*. New Brunswick, NJ: Rutgers University Press.

Johnson, E. A. (1976). *To the first Americans: The sixth report on the Indian health program of the U.S. Public Health Service*. Washington, DC: DHEW Publication (HSA) 77–1000.

Jonas, S., & Kovner, A. R. (Eds.). (1998). *Health care delivery in the United States*. New York: Springer.

Jordan, B., & Heardon, S. (1979). *Barbara Jordan: A self-portrait*. Garden City, NY: Doubleday.

Jung, C. G. (Ed.). (1964). *Man and his symbols*. Garden City, NY: Doubleday.

Kain, J. F. (Ed.). (1969). *Race and poverty: The economics of discrimination*. Englewood Cliffs, NJ: Prentice Hall.

Kanellos, N. (1997). *Hispanic firsts*. Detroit: Visible Ink.

Kaptchuk, T., & Croucher, M. (1987). *The healing arts*. New York: Summit Books.

Karolevitz, R. F. (1967). *Doctors of the old west*. New York: Bonanza Books.

Katz, J. H. (1978). *White awareness*. Norman: University of Oklahoma Press.

Kaufman, B. N., & Kaufman, S. L. (1982). *A land beyond tears*. Garden City, NY: Doubleday.

Kavanagh, K. H., & Kennedy, P. H. (1992). *Promoting cultural diversity: Strategies for health care professionals*. Newbury Park, CA: Sage.

Keith, J. (1982). *Old people as people: Social and cultural influences on aging and old age*. Boston, MA: Little, Brown.

Keith, J. (1982). *Old people, new lives*. Chicago: The University of Chicago Press.

Kekahbah, J., & Wood, R. (Eds.). (1980). *Life cycle of the American Indian family*. Norman, OK: AIANA Publishing Co.

Kelly, I. (1965). *Folk practice in North Mexico: Birth customs, folk medicine, and spiritualism in the Laguna Zone*. Austin: University of Texas Press.

Kelsey, M. T. (1973). *Healing and Christianity*. New York: Harper & Row.

Kennedy, E. M. (1972). *In critical condition: The crises in America's health care*. New York: Simon & Schuster.

Kennett, F. (1976). *Folk medicine, fact and fiction*. New York: Crescent Books.

Kiev, A. (1968). *Curanderismo: Mexican-American folk psychiatry*. New York: Free Press.

Kiev, A. (1964). *Magic, faith and healing: Studies in primitive psychiatry today*. New York: Free Press.

Killens, J. O. (1988). *The cotillion*. New York: Ballantine.

Kilner, W. J. (1965). *The human aura*. Secaucus, NJ: Citadel Press.

Kincaid, J. (1988). *A small place*. New York: Farrar, Straus and Giroux.

King, D. H. (1988). *Cherokee heritage*. Cherokee, NC: Cherokee Communications.

Kingston, M. H. (1989). *Tripmaster monkey: His fake book*. New York: Knopf.

Kirkland, J., Matthews, H. F. M., Sullivan, C. W., III, et al. (Eds.). (1992). *Herbal and magical medicine: Traditional healing today*. Durham, NC: Duke University Press.

Klein, A. M. (1991). *Sugarball, the American game, the Dominican dream*. New Haven, CT: Yale University Press.

Klein, J. W. (1980). *Jewish identity and self-esteem: Healing wounds through ethnotherapy*. New York: Institute on Pluralism and Group Identity.

Klein, M. (1998). *A time to be born: Customs and folklore of Jewish birth*. Philadelphia, PA: Jewish Publication Society.

Kluckhohn, C. (1944). *Navaho witchcraft*. Boston: Beacon Press.

Kluckhohn, C., & Leighton, D. (1962). *The Navaho* (rev. ed.). Garden City, NY: Doubleday and Co.

Kmit, A., Luciow, L. L., Luciow, J., et al. (1979). *Ukrainian Easter eggs and how we make them*. Minneapolis, MN: Ukrainian Gift Shop.

Knudtson, P., & Suzuki, D. (1992). *Wisdom of the elders*. Toronto: Stoddart.

Knutson, A. L. (1965). *The individual, society, and health behavior*. New York: Russell Sage Foundation.

Komisar, L. (1974). *Down and out in the USA: A history of social welfare*. New York: New Viewpoints.

Kordel, L. (1974). *Natural folk remedies*. New York: Putnam's.

Kosa, J., & Zola, I. K. (1976). *Poverty and health: A sociological analysis* (2nd ed.). Cambridge, MA: Harvard University Press.

Kotelchuck, D. (Ed.). (1976). *Prognosis negative*. New York: Vintage Books.

Kotz, N. (1971). *Let them eat promises*. Garden City, NY: Doubleday.

Kovner, A. (Ed.). (1990). *Health care delivery in the United States* (4th ed.). New York: Springer.

Kramer, R. M. (1969). *Participation of the poor*. Englewood Cliffs, NJ: Prentice Hall.

Kraut, A. M. (1994). *Silent travelers: Germs, genes, and the immigrant menace*. New York: Basic Books.

Kraybeill, D. B. (1989). *The riddle of Amish culture*. Baltimore: Johns Hopkins.

Kreiger, D. (1979). *The therapeutic touch*. Englewood Cliffs, NJ: Prentice Hall.

Krippner, S., & Villaldo, A. (1976). *The realms of healing*. Millbrae, CA: Celestial Arts.

Kronenfeld, J. J. (1993). *Controversial issues in health care policy*. Newbury Park, CA: Sage.

Kunitz, S. J., & Levy, J. E. (1991). *Navajo aging: The transition from family to institutional support*. Tucson: University of Arizona Press.

Lake, M. G. (1991). *Native healer initiation into an art*. Wheaton, IL: Quest Books.

Landmann, R. S. (Ed.). (1981). *The problem of the undocumented worker*. Albuquerque: Latin American Institute, University of New Mexico.

Lasker, R. D. (1997). *Medicine and public health*. New York: New York Academy of Medicine.

Lassiter, S. (1995). *Multicultural clients*. Westport, CT: Greenwood.

Last, J. M. (1987). *Public health and human ecology*. Norwalk, CT: Appleton.

Lau, T. (1979). *The handbook of Chinese horoscopes*. Philadelphia: Harper & Row.

Lavelle, R. (Ed.). (1995). *America's new war on poverty: A reader for action*. San Francisco: KQED Books.

Lawless, E. J. (1988). *God's peculiar people*. Lexington: University of Kentucky Press.

Lee, P. R., & Estes, C. L. (Eds.). (1994). *The nation's health* (4th ed.). Boston, MA: Jones & Bartlett.

Leek, S. (1975). *Herbs: Medicine and mysticism*. Chicago: Henry Regnery.

Leff, S., & Leff, V. (1957). *From witchcraft to world health*. New York: Macmillan.

Leininger, M. (1970). *Nursing and anthropology: Two worlds to blend*. New York: Wiley.

Leininger, M. (1978). *Transcultural nursing: Concepts, theories, and practices*. New York: Wiley.

Leong, L. (1974). *Acupuncture: A layman's view*. New York: Signet.

Lerner, M. (1994). *Choices in healing*. Cambridge: MIT Press.

Leslau, C., & Leslau, W. (1985). *African proverbs*. White Plains, NY: Peter Pauper Press.

Lesnoff-Caravaglia, G. (Ed.). (1987). *Realistic expectations for long life*. New York: Human Sciences Press.

Lewis, O. (1966). *A death in the Sanchez family*. New York: Random House.

Lewis, O. (1959). *Five families: Mexican case studies in the culture of poverty*. New York: New American Library Basic Books.

Lewis, O. (1966). *La vida: A Puerto Rican family in the culture of poverty—San Juan and New York*. New York: Random House.

Lewis, O. (1961). *The children of Sanchez: Autobiography of a Mexican family*. New York: Random House.

Lewis, T. H. (1990). *The medicine men: Oglala Sioux ceremony and healing*. Lincoln: University of Nebraska Press.

Lich, G. E. (1981). *The German Texans*. San Antonio, TX: The Institute of Texan Cultures.

Lieban, R. W. (1967). *Cebuano sorcery.* Berkeley: University of California Press.

Linck, E. S., & Roach J. G. (1989). *Eats: A Folkhistory of Texas foods.* Fort Worth: Texas Christian University Press.

Lipson, J. G., Dibble, S. L., & Minarik, P. A. (1996). *Culture and nursing care: A pocket guide.* San Francisco: UCSF Nursing Press.

Litoff, J. B. (1978). *American midwives 1860 to the present.* Westport, CT: Greenwood Press.

LittleDog, P. (1994). *Border healing woman: The story of Jewel Babb* (2nd ed.). Austin: University of Texas Press.

Livingston, I. L. (Ed.). (1994). *Handbook of black American health.* Westport, CT: Greenwood Press.

Logan, P. (1981). *Irish country cures.* Dublin: Talbot Press.

Louv, R. (1980). *Southwind: The Mexican migration.* San Diego: San Diego Union, 1980.

Lovering, A. T. (1923). *The household physician.* Vols. 1 & 2. Boston, MA: Woodruff.

Lum, D. (1992). *Social work practice and people of color: A process-stage approach* (2nd ed.). Pacific Grove, CA: Brooks/Cole.

Lynch, L. R. (Ed.). (1969). *The cross-cultural approach to health behavior.* Rutherford, NJ: Fairleigh Dickenson University Press.

Lyon, W. S. (1996). *Encyclopedia of Native American healing.* New York: Norton.

Mackintosh, J. (1836). *Principles of pathology and practice of physics* (3rd ed.) Vol. 1. Philadelphia, PA: Key & Biddle.

MacNutt, F. (1974). *Healing.* Notre Dame, IN: Ave Maria Press.

MacNutt, F. (1977). *The power to heal.* Notre Dame, IN: Ave Maria Press.

Magida, A. J. (Ed.). (1996). *How to be a perfect stranger,* Vol. 1. Woodstock, VT: Jewish Lights Publishing.

Malinowski, B. (1956). *Magic, science, and religion.* Garden City, NY: Doubleday.

Maloney, C. (Ed.). (1976). *The evil eye.* New York: Columbia University Press.

Malpezzi, F. M., & Clement, W. M. (1992). *Italian American folklore.* Little Rock, AR: August House Publishers.

Mandell, B. R. (Ed.). (1975). *Welfare in America: Controlling the "dangerous classes."* Englewood Cliffs, NJ: Prentice Hall.

Manderschied, R. W., & Sonnenschein, M. A. (Eds.). (1992). *Mental health, United States, 1992.* Washington, DC: Center for Mental Health Services and National Institute of Mental Health. Government Printing Office, DHHS Pub. No. (SMA) 92-1942, 1992.

Mann, F. (1972). Acupuncture: *The Ancient Chinese art of healing and how it works scientifically.* New York: Vintage Books.

Marquez, G. G. (1998). *Love in the time of cholera.* New York: Alfred A. Knopf.

Marsella, A. B., & Pedersens, P. B. (Eds.). 1982 *Cross cultural counseling and psychotherapy.* New York: Pergamon.

Marsella, A. J., & White, G. M. (Eds.). (1982). *Cultural conceptions of mental health therapy.* London: D. Reidel.

Martin, J., & Todnem, A. (1984). *Cream and bread.* Hastings, MN: Redbird Productions.

Martin, J. L., & Nelson, S. J. (1994). *They glorified Mary, we glorified rice.* Hastings, MN: Caragana Press.

Martin, J. L. (1995). *They had stories, we had chores.* Hastings, MN: Caragana Press.

Martin, L. C. (1984). *Wildflower folklore.* Charlotte, NC: East Woods Press.

Martinez, R. A. (Ed.). (1978). *Hispanic culture and health care.* St. Louis, MO: C. V. Mosby.

Matlins, S. M., & Magida, A. J. (Eds.). (1997). *How to be a perfect stranger,* Vol. 2. Woodstock, VT: Jewish Lights Publishing.

Matsumoto M. (1988). *The unspoken way.* Tokyo: Kodansha International.

Matthiessen, P. (1980). *In the spirit of Crazy Horse.* New York: Viking Press.

McBrid, I. R. (1975). *Practical folk medicine of Hawaii.* Hilo: Petroglyph Press.

McBride, J. (1996). *The color of water.* New York: Riverhead Books.

McCall, N. (1995). *Makes me wanna holler.* New York: Vintage Books.

McClain, M. (1988). *A feeling for life: Cultural identity, community, and the arts.* Chicago: Urban Traditions.

McCubbin, H. I., Thompson, E. A., Thompson, A. I., et al. (1994). *Resiliency in ethnic minority families.* Vol. 1, *Native and immigrant American families.* Madison: WI: University of Wisconsin.

McCubbin, H., Thompson, E. A., Thompson, A. I., et al. (1995). *Resiliency in ethnic minority families.* Vol. 2, *African-American families.* Madison: University of Wisconsin Center.

McCubbin, H. I., Thompson, E. A., Thompson, A. I., et al. (1994). *Sense of coherence and resiliency.* Madison: University of Wisconsin.

McGill, O. (1977). *The mysticism and magic of India.* South Brunswick, NJ, and New York: A. S. Baines.

McGoldrick, M., Giordano, J., & Pearce, J. K. (1996). *Ethnicity and family therapy* (2nd ed.). New York: Guilford Press.

McGregor, J. H. (1940). *The Wounded Knee massacre from the viewpoint of the Sioux.* Rapid City, SD: Fenwyn Press.

McLary, K. (1993). *Amish style.* Bloomington: Indiana Press.

McLemore, S. D. (1980). *Racial and ethnic relations in America.* Boston, MA: Allyn & Bacon.

Means, R. (1995). *Where white men fear to tread.* New York: St. Martin's Press.

Mechanic, D. (1968). *Medical sociology: A selective view.* New York: Free Press.

Melton, J. G. (2000). *American religions.* Santa Barbara, CA: A B C Clio.

Melville, H. (1851). *Moby Dick* (1967 edition). New York: Bantam Books.

Menchu, R. (1983). *I, Rigoberta Menchu.* Trans. A. Wright. London: Verso.

Merrill, F. E. (1962). *Society and culture.* Englewood Cliffs, NJ: Prentice Hall.

Metraux, A. (1972). *Voodoo in Haiti.* New York: Schocken Books.

Meyer, C. E. (1985). *American folk medicine.* Glenwood, IL: Meyerbooks.

Micozzi, M. S. (1996). *Fundamentals of complementary and alternative medicine.* New York: Churchill.

Milio, N. (1975). *The care of health in communities: Access for outcasts.* New York: Macmillan.

Millman, M. (1977). *The unkindest cut.* New York: William Morrow.

Mindel, C. H., & Habenstein, R. W. (Eds.). (1976). *Ethnic families in America.* New York: Elsevier.

Miner, H. (1939). *St. Denis, a French Canadian parish.* Chicago: University of Chicago Press.

Moldenke, H. N., & Moldenke, A. L. (1952). *Plants of the Bible.* New York: Dover Publications.

Montagu, A. (1971). *Touching.* New York: Harper & Row.

Montgomery, R. (1973). *Born to heal.* New York: Coward, McCann, and Geoghegan.

Moody, R. A. (1976). *Life after life.* New York: Bantam.

Mooney, J. (1982). *Myths of the Cherokee and sacred formulas of the Cherokees.* Nashville, TN: Charles and Randy Elder—Booksellers, and

Cherokee, NC: Museum of the Cherokee Indian.

Morgan, M. (1991). *Mutant message downunder*. Lees Summit, MO: MM CO.

Morgenstern, J. (1966). *Rites of birth, marriage, death, and kindred occasions among the Semites*. Chicago: Quadrangle Books.

Morley, P., & Wallis, R. (Eds.). (1978). *Culture and curing*. Pittsburgh: University of Pittsburgh Press.

Morrison, T. (1987). *Beloved*. New York: Knopf/Random House.

Morrison, T. (1981). *Tar baby*. New York: Alfred A. Knopf.

Morton, L. T., & Moore, R. J. (1998). *A chronology of medicine and related sciences*. Cambridge: University Press, 1998.

Murray, P. (1987). *Song in a weary throat: An American pilgrimage*. New York: Harper & Row.

Mushkin, S. V. (1974). *Consumer incentives for health care*. New York: Prodist.

National Center for Health Statistics. (1998). *Health United States 1998 with socioeconomic status and health chartbook*. Hyattsville, MD: Author.

Neihardt, J. G. (1991—original 1951). *When the tree flowered*. Lincoln: University of Nebraska Press.

Neihardt, J. G. (1998—original 1961). *Black Elk speaks*. Lincoln: University of Nebraska Press.

Neihardt, N. (1993). *The sacred hoop*. Tekamah, NE: Neihardt.

Nelli, H. S. (1983). *From immigrants to ethnics: The Italian Americans*. Oxford: Oxford University Press.

Nelson, D. (1985). *Food combining simplified*. Santa Cruz, CA: The Plan.

Nemetz-Robinson, G. L. (1988). *Crosscultural understanding*. New York: Prentice Hall.

Nerburn, K., & Mengelkoch, L. (Eds.). (1991). *Native American wisdom*. San Rafael, CA: New World Library.

Neugrossschel, J. (1991). *Great tales of Jewish occult and fantasy*. New York: Wings Books.

Newman, K. D. (1975). *Ethnic American short stories*. New York: Pocket Books.

Noble, M. (1997). *Sweet grass lives of contemporary Native women of the Northeast*. Mashpee, MA: C. J. Mills.

Norman, J. C. (Ed.). (1969). *Medicine in the ghetto*. New York: Appleton-Century-Crofts.

North, J. H., & Grodsky, S. J. (Comp.). (1979). *Immigration literature: Abstracts of demographic, economic, and policy studies*. Washington, DC: U.S. Department of Justice, Immigration & Naturalization Service.

Novak, M. (1972). *The rise of the unmeltable ethnics*. New York: Macmillan.

Null, G., & Stone, C. (1976). *The Italian-Americans*. Harrisburg, PA: Stackpole Books.

O'Berennan, J., & Smith, N. (1981). *The crystal icon*. Austin, TX: Galahad Press.

Oduyoye, M. (1996). *Words and meaning in Yoruba religion*. London: Karnak House.

Opler, M. K. (Ed.). (1959). *Culture and mental health*. New York: Macmillan.

Orlando, L. (1993). *The multicultural game book*. New York: Scholastic Professional Books.

Orque, M. S., Block, B., & Monrray, L. S. A. (1983). *Ethnic nursing care: A Multicultural approach*. St. Louis, MO: C. V. Mosby.

Osofsky, G. (1963). Harlem: *The making of a ghetto*. New York: Harper & Row.

Overfield, T. (1985). *Biologic variation in health and illness*. Menlo Park, CA: Addison-Wesley.

Ozaniec, N. (1997). *Little book of Egyptian wisdom*. Rockport, MA: Element.

Padilla, E. (1958). *Up from Puerto Rico*. New York: Columbia University Press.

Paley, V. G. (1979). *White teacher*. Cambridge, MA: Harvard University Press.

Palos, S. (1971). *The Chinese art of healing*. New York: Herter and Herter.

Pappworth, M. H. (1967). *Human guinea pigs: Experimentation on man*. Boston, MA: Beacon Press.

Parsons, T., & Clark, K. B. (1965). *The Negro American*. Boston, MA: Beacon Press.

Paul, B. (Ed.). (1955). *Health, culture, and community: Case studies of public reactions to health programs*. New York: Russell Sage Foundation.

Payer, L. (1988). *Medicine and culture*. New York: Penguin Books.

Pearsall, M. (1963). *Medical behavior science: A selected bibliography of cultural anthropology, social psychology, and sociology in medicine*. Louisville: University of Kentucky Press.

Peltier, L. (1999). *Prison writings: My life is my sun dance*. New York: St. Martin's Press.

Pelto, P. J., & Pelto, G. H. (1978). *Anthropological research: The structure of inquiry* (2nd ed.). Cambridge: Cambridge University Press.

Pelton, R. W. (1973). *Voodoo charms and talismans*. New York: Popular Library.

Perera, V. (1995). *The cross and the pear tree*. Berkeley: University of California Press.

Petry, A. (1985). *The street*. Boston: Beacon Press.

Philpott, L. L. (1979). "A Descriptive Study of Birth Practices and Midwifery in the Lower Rio Grande Valley of Texas." Ph.D. diss., University of Texas Health Science Center at Houston School of Public Health.

Pierce, R. V. (1983). *The people's common sense medical advisor in plain English, or medicine simplified* (12th ed.). Buffalo, NY: World's Dispensary.

Piven, F. F., & Cloward, R. A. (1971). *Regulating the poor: The functions of public welfare*. New York: Vintage Books.

Plotkin, M. J. (1993). *Tales of a shaman's apprentice*. New York: Viking.

Popenoe, C. (1977). *Wellness*. Washington, DC: YES!

Powell, C. A. (1938). *Bound feet*. Boston: Warren Press.

Power, S. (1994). *The grass dancer*. New York: Putnam.

Prabhupada, A. C. (1970). *Bhaktivedanta Swami. KRSNA: The supreme personality of godhead*. Vol. 1. Los Angeles: The Bhaktivedanta Book Trust.

Prose, F. (1977). *Marie Laveau*. New York: Berkeley.

Proulx, E. A. (1996). *Accordion crimes*. New York: Scribner.

Purnell, L. D., & Paulanka, B. J. (1988). *Transcultural health care*. Philadelphia: F. A. Davis.

Rand, C. *The Puerto Ricans*. (1958). New York: Oxford University Press.

Read, M. (1966). *Culture, Health, and Disease*. London: Javistock Publications, 1966.

Rector-Page, L. G. (1992). *Healthy healing: An alternative healing reference* (9th ed.). San Fransisco, CA: Healthy Healing Publications.

Redman, E. (1973). *The dance of legislation*. New York: Simon & Schuster.

Reichard, G. A. (1977). *Navajo medicine-man sandpaintings*. New York: Dover.

Reneaux, J. J. (1992). *Cajun folktales*. Little Rock, AR: August House Publishers.

Rist, R. C. (1979). *Desegregated schools: Appraisals of an American experiment.* New York: Academic Press.

Riva, A. (1990). *Devotions to the saints.* Los Angeles: International Imports.

Riva, A. (1985). *Magic with incense and powders.* N. Hollywood, CA: International Imports, 1985.

Riva, A. (1974). *The modern herbal spellbook.* N. Hollywood, CA: International Imports.

Rivera, J. R. (1977). *Puerto Rican tales.* Mayaquez, Puerto Rico: Ediciones Libero.

Roby, P. (Ed.). (1974). *The poverty establishment.* Englewood Cliffs, NJ: Prentice Hall.

Rodriquez, C. E. (1991). *Puerto Ricans born in the U.S.A.* Boulder, CO: Westview Press.

Roemer, M. I. (1990). *An introduction to the U.S. health care system* (2nd ed.). New York: Springer.

Rogler, L. H. (1972). *Migrant in the city.* New York: Basic Books.

Rohde, E. S. (1922, 1971). *The Old English herbs.* New York: Dover.

Rose, P. I. (1981). *They and we: Racial and ethnic relations in the United States* (3rd ed.). New York: Random House.

Rosen, P. (1980). *The neglected dimension: Ethnicity in American life.* Notre Dame, London: University of Notre Dame Press.

Rosenbaum, B. Z. (1985). *How to avoid the evil eye.* New York: St. Martin's Press.

Ross, N. W. (1960). *The World of Zen.* New York: Vintage Books.

Rossbach, S. (1987). *Interior design with feng shui.* New York: Arkana.

Roter, D. L., & Hall, J. A. (1993). *Doctors talking with patients.* Westport, CT: Auburn House.

Rude, D. (Ed.). (1972). *Alienation: Minority groups.* New York: Wiley.

Russell, A. J. (1937). *Health in his wings.* London: Metheun.

Ryan, W. (1971). *Blaming the victim.* New York: Vintage Books.

S., E. M. (1927). *The house of wonder: A romance of psychic healing.* London: Rider.

Santillo, H. (1983). *Herbal combinations from authoritative sources.* Provo, UT: NuLife.

Santino, J. (1994). *All around the year.* Chicago: University of Illinois Press.

Santoli, A. (1988). *New Americans.* New York: Ballantine.

Sargent, D. A. (1904). *Health, strength, and power.* New York: HM Caldwell.

Saunders, L. (1954). *Cultural difference and medical care: The case of the Spanish-speaking people of the Southwest.* New York: Russell Sage Foundation.

Saunders, R. (1927). *Healing through the spirit agency.* London: Hutchinson.

Schneider, M. (1987). *Self healing: My life and vision.* New York: Routledge & Kegan Paul.

Scholem, G. G. (1941). *Major trends in Jewish mysticism.* New York: Schocken Books.

School, B. F. (1924). *Library of health complete guide to prevention and cure of disease.* Philadelphia, PA: Historical.

Schrefer, S. (Ed.). (1994). *Quick reference to cultural assessment.* St. Louis, MO: Mosby.

Scott, W. R., & Volkart, E. H. (1966). *Medical care.* New York: Wiley.

Senior, C. (1961). *The Puerto Ricans, strangers—then neighbors.* Chicago: Quadrangle Books.

Serinus, J. (Ed.). (1986). *Psychoimmunity and the healing process.* Berkeley, CA: Celestial Arts.

Sexton, P. C. (1965). *Spanish Harlem.* New York: Harper & Row.

Shaw, W. (1975). *Aspects of Malaysian magic.* Kuala Lumpur, Malaysia: Naziabum. Nigara.

Sheinkin, D. (1986). *Path of the Kabbalah.* New York: Paragon House.

Shelton, F. (1965). *Pioneer comforts and kitchen remedies: Oldtime highland secrets from the Blue Ridge and Great*

Smoky Mountains. High Point, NC: Hutcraft.

Shelton, F. (Ed.). (1969). *Pioneer superstitions*. High Point, NC: Hutcraft.

Shenkin, B. N. (1974). *Health care for migrant workers: Policies and politics*. Cambridge, MA: Ballinger.

Shepard, R. F., & Levi, V. G. (1982). *Live and be well*. New York: Ballantine Books.

Shih-Chen, L. (1973). *Chinese medicinal herbs*. Trans. F. P. Smith & G. A. Stuart. San Francisco: Georgetown Press.

Shor, I. (1986). *Culture wars: School and society in the conservative restoration 1969–1984*. Boston, MA: Routledge & Kegan Paul.

Shorter, E. (1987). *The health century*. New York: Doubleday.

Shostak, A. B., Van Til, J., & Van Til, S. B. (1973). *Privilege in America: An end to inequality?* Englewood Cliffs, NJ: Prentice Hall.

Silver, G. (1976). *A spy in the house of medicine*. Germantown, MD: Aspen Systems Corp.

Silverman, D. (1989). *Legends of Safed*. Jerusalem: Gefen.

Silverstein, M. E., Chang, I-L., & Macon, N., trans. (1975). *Acupuncture and moxibustion*. New York: Schocken Books.

Simmen, E. (Ed.). (1972). *Pain and promise: The Chicano today*. New York: New American Library.

Simmons, A. G. (n.d.). *A witch's brew*. Coventry, CT: Caprilands Herb Farm.

Skelton, R. (1985). *Talismanic magic*. York Beach, ME: Samuel Weiser.

Slater, P. (1970). *The pursuit of loneliness*. Boston: Beacon Press.

Smith, H. (1958). *The religions of man*. New York: Harper & Row.

Smith, L. (1963). *Killers of the dream*. Garden City, NY: Doubleday.

Smith, P. (1962). *The origins of modern culture, 1543–1687*. New York: Collier Books.

Sowell, T. (1981). *Ethnic America*. New York: Basic Books.

Sowell, T. (1996). *Migrations and cultures*. New York: Basic Books.

Spann, M. B. (1992). *Literature-based multicultural activities*. New York: Scholastic Professional Books.

Spector, R. E. (1983). "A Description of the Impact of Medicare on Health-Illness Beliefs and Practices of White Ethnic Senior Citizens in Central Texas." Ph.D. diss., University of Texas at Austin School of Nursing, 1983; Ann Arbor, MI: University Microfilms International.

Spector, R. E. (1998). *CulturalCare: Maternal infant issues*. Baltimore: Williams & Wilkins (video).

Spicer, E. (Ed.). (1977). *Ethnic medicine in the Southwest*. New York: Russell Sage Foundation.

Stack, C. B. (1974). *All our kin*. New York: Harper & Row.

Starr, P. (1982). *The social transformation of American medicine*. New York: Basic Books.

Steele, J. D. (1884). *Hygienic physiology*. New York: A. S. Barnes.

Steinberg, M. (1947). *Basic Judaism*. New York: Harcourt, Brace and World.

Steinberg, S. (2001) *The ethnic myth: Race, ethnicity, and class in America*. Boston, MA: Beacon Press.

Steiner, S. (1969). *La Raza: The Mexican Americans*. New York: Harper & Row.

Steinsaltz, A. (1980). *The thirteen petalled rose*. New York: Basic Books.

Stephan, W. G., & Feagin, J. R. (1980). *School desegregation past, present, future*. New York: Plenum.

Stevens, A. (1974). *Vitamins and remedies*. High Point, NC: Hutcraft.

Stewart, J. (Ed.). (1973). *Bridges not walls*. Reading, MA: Addison-Wesley.

Still, C. E., Jr. (1991). *Frontier doctor medical pioneer*. Kirksville, MO: Thomas Jefferson University Press.

Stoll, R. I. (1990). *Concepts in nursing: A Christian perspective*. Madison,

WI: Intervarsity Christian Fellowship.

Stone, E. (1962). *Medicine among the American Indians.* New York: Hafner.

Storlie, F. (1970). *Nursing and the social conscience.* New York: Appleton-Century-Crofts.

Storm, H. (1972). *Seven arrows.* New York: Ballantine Books.

Strauss, A., & Corbin, J. M. (1988). *Shaping a new health care system.* San Francisco: Jossey-Bass.

Styron, W. (1966). *The confessions of Nat Turner.* New York: Random House.

Swazey, J. P., & Reeds, K. (1978). *Today's medicine, tomorrow's science.* Washington, DC: U.S. Government Department of Health, Education, and Welfare.

Sweet, M. (1976). *Common edible plants of the west.* Happy Camp, CA: Naturegraph.

Szasz, T. S. (1961). *The myth of mental illness.* New York: Dell.

Takaki, R. (1993). *A different mirror: A history of multicultural America.* Boston, MA: Little, Brown.

Tallant, R. (1946). *Voodoo in New Orleans.* New York: Collier Books.

Tan, A. (1989). *The Joy Luck Club.* New York: Ivy Books.

Tan, A. (2001). *The bonesetter's daughter.* New York: Putnam & Sons.

Te Selle, S. (Ed.). (1973). *The rediscovery of ethnicity: Its implications for culture and politics in America.* New York: Harper & Row.

ten Boom, C. (1971). *The hiding place.* Washington Depot, CT: Chosen Books.

Thernstrom, S. (Ed.). (1980). *Harvard encyclopedia of American ethnic groups.* Cambridge: Harvard University Press.

Thomas, C. (1983). *They came to Pittsburgh.* Pittsburgh: Post-Gazette.

Thomas, P. (1958). *Down these mean streets.* New York: Signet Books.

Thomas, P. (1972). *Savior, Savior, hold my hand.* Garden City, NY: Doubleday.

Tierra, M. (1990). *The way of herbs.* New York: Pocket Books.

Titmuss, R. M. (1971). *The gift relationship.* New York: Vintage.

Tomasi, S. M. (Ed.). (1980). *National directory of research centers, repositories, and organizations of Italian culture in the United States.* Torino: Fondazione Giovanni Agnelli.

Tompkins, P., & Bird, C. (1973). *The secret life of plants.* New York: Avon.

Tooker, E. (Ed.). (1979). *Native American spirituality of the eastern woodlands.* New York: Paulist Press.

Torres, E. (1982). *Green medicine: Traditional Mexican-American herbal remedies.* Kingsville, TX: Nieves Press.

Torres-Gill, F. M. (1982). *Politics of aging among elder Hispanics.* Washington, DC: University Press of America.

Touchstone, S. J. (1983). *Herbal and folk medicine of Louisiana and adjacent states.* Princeton, LA: Folk-Life Books.

Trachtenberg, J. (1939). *Jewish magic and superstition.* New York: Behrman House.

Trachtenberg, J. (1983). *The devil and the Jews.* Philadelphia, PA: The Jewish Publication Society of America. (Original publication, New Haven, CT: Yale University Press, 1945.)

Trattner, W. I. (1974). *From poor law to welfare state: A history of social welfare in America.* New York: Free Press.

Trotter, R., II, & Chavira, J. A. (1981). *Curanderismo: Mexican American folk healing.* Athens, GA: University of Georgia Press.

Tucker, G. H. (1977). *Virginia supernatural tales.* Norfolk, VA: Donning.

Tula, M. T. (1994). *Hear my testimony.* Boston, MA: South End Press.

Twining, M. A., & Baird, K. E. (Eds.). (1991). *Sea Island Roots: African presence in the Carolinas and Georgia.* Trenton, NJ: Africa World Press.

Unger, S. (Ed.). (1977). *The destruction of American Indian families.* New York: Association on American Indian Affairs.

U.S. Commission on Civil Rights. (1976). *Fulfilling the letter and spirit of the law.* Washington, DC: Government Printing Office.

U. S. Commission on Civil Rights. (1970). *Mexican Americans and the administration of justice in the Southwest.* Washington, DC: Government Printing Office.

U.S. Department of Commerce, Bureau of the Census. (1980). *Ancestry of the population by State: 1980.* Washington, DC: Government Printing Office.

U. S. Department of Commerce, Bureau of the Census. (1982, September). *Population profile of the United States: 1981.* "Population Characteristics," ser. 20, no. 374.

U.S. Department of Health and Human Services. (1997). *Comprehensive health care program for American Indians and Alaska Natives.* Rockville, MD: Public Health Service, Indian Health Service.

U. S. Department of Health and Human Services. (1997). *Regional differences in Indian health.* Rockville, MD: Public Health Service, Indian Health Service.

U. S. Department of Health and Human Services. (1997). *Trends in Indian Health.* Rockville, MD: Public Health Service, Indian Health Service.

U. S. Department of Health and Human Services. (1993). *Health United States 1992 and healthy people 2000 review.* Washington, DC: United States Department of Health

and Human Services, Public Health Service Centers for Disease Control and Prevention. DHHS Pub. No. (PHS) 93-1232.

U. S. Department of Health and Human Services. (1992). *Healthy people 2000 national health promotion and disease prevention objectives: Full report with commentary.* Boston: Jones and Bartlett.

U.S. Department of Health, Education, and Welfare. *Health in America: 1776–1976.* Washington, DC: DHEW pub. (HRA) 76-616, 1976.

U.S. Department of Justice, Immigration and Naturalization Service. (1979). *Immigration literature: Abstracts of demographic economic and policy studies.* Washington, DC: Government Printing Office.

Valentine, C. A. (1968). *Culture and poverty.* Chicago: University of Chicago Press.

Wade, M. (1946). *The French-Canadian outlook.* New York: Viking Press.

Wade, M. (1955). *The French-Canadians, 1876–1945.* New York: Macmillan.

Walker, A. (1994). *The temple of my familiar.* New York: Harcourt, Brace, Jovanovich.

Wall, S. (1994). *Shadowcatchers.* New York: HarperCollins.

Wall, S., & Arden, H. (1990). *Wisdomkeepers meetings with native American spiritual elders.* Hillsboro, OR: Beyond Words Publishing Co.

Wallace, R. B. (Ed.). *Public health and preventive medicine* (14th ed.). Stamford, CT: Appleton & Lange.

Wallnöfer, H., & von Rottauscher, A. (1972). *Chinese folk medicine.* Trans. M. Palmedo. New York: New American Library.

Warner, D. (1979). *The Health of Mexican Americans in South Texas.* Austin, TX: Lyndon Baines Johnson School of Public Affairs, University of Texas at Austin.

Warner, D., & Red, K. (1993). *Health care across the border.* Austin, TX: LBJ School.

Warren, N. (Ed.). (1980). *Studies in cross-cultural psychology.* New York: Academic Press.

Weible, W. (1983). *Medjugore: The message.* Orleans, MA: Paraclete Press.

Wei-kang, F. (1975). *The story of Chinese acupuncture and moxibustion.* Peking: Foreign Languages Press.

Weil, A. (1983). *Health and healing.* Boston, MA: Houghton Mifflin.

Weinbach, S. (1991). *Rabbenu Yisrael Abuchatzira: The story of his life and wonders.* Brooklyn, NY: ASABA-FUJIE publication.

Weinberg, R. D. (1967). *Eligibility for entry to the United States of America.* Dobbs Ferry, NY: Oceana.

Wiebe, R., & Johnson, Y. (1998). *Stolen life—The journey of a Cree woman.* Athens: Ohio University Press.

Weiss, G., & Weiss, S. (1985). *Growing and using the healing herbs.* New York: Wings Books.

Wheelwright, E. G. (1974). *Medicinal plants and their history.* New York: Dover.

Wilen, J., & Wilen, L. (1984). *Chicken soup and other folk remedies.* New York: Fawcett Columbine.

Williams, R. A. (Ed.). (1975). *Textbook of black-related diseases.* New York: McGraw-Hill.

Williams, S. J., & Torrens, P. R. (1990). *Introduction to health services* (3rd ed.). New York: Wiley.

Wilson, F. A., & Neuhauser, D. (1982). *Health services in the United States* (2nd ed.). Cambridge, MA: Ballinger.

Wilson, S. G. (1992). *The drummer's path: Moving the spirit with ritual and traditional drumming.* Rochester, VT: Destiny Books.

Winkler, G. (1981). *Dybbuk.* New York: Judaica Press.

Wolfson, E. (1993). *From the earth to the sky.* Boston, MA: Houghton Mifflin.

Wright, E. (1984). *The book of magical talismans.* Minneapolis, MN: Marlar Publishing, Co.

Wright, R. (1937). *Black boy.* New York: Harper & Brothers.

Wright, R. (1940). *Native son.* New York: Grosset & Dunlop.

Wright-Hybbard, E. (1977–1992). *A brief study course in homeopathy.* Philadelphia: Formur.

Yambura, B. S. (1960). *A change and a parting.* Ames: University of Iowa Press.

Young, J. H. (1967). *The medical messiahs.* Princeton, NJ: Princeton University Press.

Zambrana, R. E. (Ed.). (1982). *Work, family, and health: Latina women in transition.* New York: Fordham University.

Zborowski, M. (1969). *People in pain.* San Francisco: Jossey-Bass.

Zeitlin, S. J., Kotkin, A. J., & Baker, H. C. (1977). *A celebration of American family folklore: Tales and traditions from the Smithsonian collection.* New York: Pantheon Books.

Zolla, E. (1969). *The writer and the shaman.* New York: Harcourt Brace Jovanovich.

Zook, J. (1972). *Exploring the secrets of treating deaf-mutes.* Peking: Foreign Languages Press.

Zook, J. (1899). *Oneida, The people of the stone.* The Church's Mission to the Oneidas. Oneida Indian Reservation, WI.

Zook, J. (1972). *Your new life in the United States.* Washington, DC: Center for Applied Linguistics.

Zook, J., & Zook, J. (1978). *Hexology.* Paradise, PA: Zook.

Index